# Opioid-Induced Hyperalgesia

# Opioid-Induced Hyperalgesia

Edited by
## Jianren Mao
*Massachusetts General Hospital*
*Harvard Medical School*
*Boston, Massachusetts, USA*

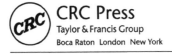

CRC Press
Taylor & Francis Group
Boca Raton  London  New York

CRC Press is an imprint of the
Taylor & Francis Group, an **informa** business

CRC Press
Taylor & Francis Group
6000 Broken Sound Parkway NW, Suite 300
Boca Raton, FL 33487-2742

First issued in paperback 2017

ISBN-13: 978-1-4200-8899-1 (hbk)
ISBN-13: 978-1-138-11270-4 (pbk)

| Library of Congress Cataloging-in-Publication Data |
| --- |

Opioid-induced hyperalgesia / edited by Jianren Mao.
    p. ; cm.
   Includes bibliographical references and index.
   ISBN-13: 978-1-4200-8899-1 (hardcover : alk. paper)
   ISBN-10: 1-4200-8899-8 (hardcover : alk. paper) 1. Opioids–Side effects. 2. Hyperalgesia. I. Mao, Jianren.
   [DNLM: 1. Hyperalgesia–chemically induced. 2. Analgesics, Opioid–adverse effects. 3. Analgesics, Opioid–therapeutic use. 4. Hyperalgesia–diagnosis. 5. Hyperalgesia–therapy. WL 710 O61 2009]
   RD86.O64O647 2009
   615′.7822–dc22

                              2009032140

**Visit the Informa Web site at**
**www.informa.com**

**and the Informa Healthcare Web site at**
**www.informahealthcare.com**

# Preface

Despite the extensive effort over several decades searching for new pharmacological tools for clinical pain treatment, opioid analgesics remain the mainstay of contemporary pain medicine. Opioid analgesics are extensively used for the management of both acute and chronic pain including cancer-related pain. Opioid analgesics have a number of side effects including respiratory depression, miosis, nausea, vomiting, constipation, biliary tract spasm, urinary retention, hypotension, dizziness, dysphoria, metal status change, and pruritis. However, most of these side effects are dose dependent and manageable in the clinical setting.

Other opioid-related clinical issues such as opioid tolerance, dependence, and addiction have limited the use of opioid analgesics in pain medicine, particularly for chronic pain management. More recently, both preclinical and clinical studies have shown that chronic exposure to opioid analgesics can alter the response of the central nervous system to nociceptive input leading to the increased pain sensitivity, which is often referred to as opioid-induced hyperalgesia. Both preclinical and clinical findings suggest that opioid analgesics that are intended to reduce pain may paradoxically increase pain under certain clinical conditions, calling for a new approach to managing clinical opioid therapy.

This book is intended to provide clinically oriented discussions on the diagnosis and management of opioid-induced hyperalgesia. Clinical practitioners who are currently involved or interested in pain management are intended primary readers, including such specialties as anesthesiology, pain medicine, neurology, oncology, palliative care, addiction medicine, primary care, rheumatology, and surgery.

The first chapter (by Dr Mao) provides an overview on the concept of opioid-induced hyperalgesia, followed by a focused discussion on possible cellular mechanisms of opioid-induced hyperalgesia and its relation to opioid tolerance (by Dr Ueda). The third chapter (by Drs Angst, Chu, Clark) provides readers with a thorough discussion on the clinical features of opioid-induced hyperalgesia and their impact in pain medicine. The clinical utility of quantitative sensory testing in the diagnosis of opioid-induced hyperalgesia is the focus of chapter 4 (by Dr Edwards), which gives the detailed accounts on the history, methodology, and clinical utility of quantitative sensory testing.

The clinical interaction between addiction and opioid therapy is a vitally important issue in pain medicine and addiction medicine. Chapter 5 (by Dr Ballantyne) and chapter 6 (by Drs Ling and Compton) focus on the relationship between addiction and clinical features and management of opioid-induced hyperalgesia. These two chapters provide profound details on the neurobiology, philosophy, clinical features, and clinical management of the interaction between addiction and opioid-induced hyperalgesia.

Chapters 7 and 8 present practical guidelines on the clinical diagnosis and management of opioid-induced hyperalgesia under various clinical circumstances, including primary care settings (by Dr McCarberg) and perioperative care (by Drs Crooks and Cohen). Additional approaches to managing opioid-induced hyperalgesia in other clinical circumstances are the topics of chapters 9, 10, and 11, which include discussions on the role of ketamine (by Dr Vorobeychik), opioid rotation and tapering (by Dr Smith), and adjuvant medications (by Drs Giampetro and Vorobeychik). The final chapter (by Dr Mao) summarizes clinical differential diagnosis between opioid-induced hyperalgesia and opioid tolerance and discusses future research directions on this important clinical phenomenon.

I would like to express my deep appreciation for my colleagues in this field, who have contributed to the work of this book project and/or basic science and clinical research on this important topic.

*Jianren Mao*

# Contents

# Contributors

**Martin S. Angst**   Stanford University School of Medicine, Stanford, California, U.S.A.

**Jane C. Ballantyne**   Penn Pain Medicine Center, University of Pennsylvania, Philadelphia, Pennsylvania, U.S.A.

**Larry F. Chu**   Stanford University School of Medicine, Stanford, California, U.S.A.

**J. David Clark**   Stanford University School of Medicine and Palo Alto Veterans Affairs Hospital, Palo Alto, California, U.S.A.

**Steven P. Cohen**   Pain Management Division, Johns Hopkins School of Medicine, Baltimore, Maryland and Walter Reed Army Medical Center, Washington, D.C., U.S.A.

**Peggy Compton**   School of Nursing, University of California at Los Angeles, Los Angeles, California, U.S.A.

**Matthew Crooks**   Department of Anesthesiology, Pain Management Division, David Geffen School of Medicine at UCLA, Los Angeles, California, U.S.A.

**Robert R. Edwards**   Department of Anesthesiology, Brigham and Women's Hospital, and Harvard School of Medicine, Boston, Massachusetts, U.S.A.

**David Giampetro**   Department of Anesthesiology, Penn State Milton S. Hershey Medical Center, Penn State College of Medicine, Hershey, Pennsylvania, U.S.A.

**Walter Ling**   Department of Psychiatry and Biobehavioral Sciences, David Geffen School of Medicine, University of California at Los Angeles, Los Angeles, California, U.S.A.

**Jianren Mao**   Department of Anesthesia, Critical Care, and Pain Medicine, Massachusetts General Hospital, Harvard Medical School, Boston, Massachusetts, U.S.A.

**Bill McCarberg**   Kaiser Permanente, Chronic Pain Management Program, University of California, San Diego, California, U.S.A.

**Howard S. Smith**   Department of Anesthesiology, Albany Medical College, Albany, New York, U.S.A.

**Hiroshi Ueda**   Division of Molecular Pharmacology and Neuroscience, Graduate School of Biomedical Sciences, Nagasaki University, Nagasaki, Japan

**Yakov Vorobeychik**   Department of Anesthesiology, Penn State Milton S. Hershey Medical Center, Penn State College of Medicine, Hershey, Pennsylvania, U.S.A.

# 1

# Overview on Opioid-Induced Hyperalgesia

**Jianren Mao**

*Department of Anesthesia, Critical Care, and Pain Medicine,*
*Massachusetts General Hospital, Harvard Medical School,*
*Boston Massachusetts, U.S.A.*

## INTRODUCTION

Opioids produce analgesia through a primarily inhibitory effect on the nociceptive system. To date, opioids remain the most powerful analgesics for clinical management of moderate to severe pain. Besides many known side effects of opioids such as sedation and constipation, chronic opioid exposure is associated with the development of tolerance to opioid analgesics. This process is largely due to an adaptive change of the opioid analgesic system that leads to the desensitization of opioid receptors and associated intracellular cascades.

Another consequence of chronic opioid exposure is the development of opioid dependence. A notable feature of opioid dependence is that hyperalgesia (exacerbated painful response to noxious stimulation) occurs during a precipitated opioid withdrawal. Over the past 15 years, compelling preclinical evidence has accumulated, indicating that hyperalgesia also occurs following opioid administration in the absence of overt, precipitated opioid withdrawal. A growing body of evidence suggests that the development of opioid-induced hyperalgesia is mediated through the neural mechanisms that involve changes at the cellular and neural circuit level, which interact with the mechanisms underlying the development of pathological pain such as pain induced by peripheral nerve injury. Thus, chronic

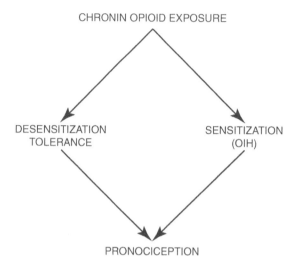

**Figure 1** Schematic illustration of two interrelated outcomes of chronic opioid exposure. Both the desensitization and sensitization processes contribute to the enhanced pronociceptive process after chronic opioid exposure.

opioid exposure also leads to a sensitization process within the central nervous system that is pronociceptive even in the presence of opioid analgesics.

As illustrated in Figure 1, the desensitization process reduces the clinical efficacy of opioid analgesics, whereas the sensitization process facilitates nociception, thereby counteracting the opioid analgesic effect. Both the desensitization and sensitization processes lead to a pronociceptive outcome that contributes to apparent clinical opioid tolerance, that is, the need for opioid dose escalation to maintain the opioid analgesic effect. Since the nociceptive system is a primitive and vital defense system, the development of analgesic tolerance and hyperalgesia in response to chronic opioid exposure helps counteract the impact of analgesics on blunting the nociceptive response as an important warning signal. This chapter will focus on preclinical evidence for opioid-induced hyperalgesia and its possible cellular mechanisms. The following chapters will discuss clinical features of opioid-induced hyperalgesia and approaches to diagnosing and managing this clinical condition. The last chapter of this book will provide a brief summary on the clinical implications of opioid-induced hyperalgesia and future research directions on this important clinical issue.

## PRECLINICAL EVIDENCE FOR OPIOID-INDUCED HYPERALGESIA

Preclinical studies of opioid tolerance assess changes of the antinociceptive efficacy before and after opioid boluses or continuous opioid administration. One of the most commonly used methods in preclinical studies is a tail-flick test, which is used to evaluate the antinociceptive effects of opioids. For example, the opioid antinociceptive effect is seen as the increased baseline nociceptive threshold in a tail-flick test. Conversely, a decrease in the baseline nociceptive threshold is an indication of the hyperalgesic response. For years, differences in baseline nociceptive thresholds before and after an opioid treatment are not readily detected using the tail-flick test, because this test often uses a steep stimulation curve with a fast-rising stimulation intensity that could mask subtle changes of a baseline nociceptive threshold. By comparison, a test that utilizes a slow-rising stimulation curve such as the foot-withdrawal test (1) enables the detection of subtle changes in baseline nociceptive threshold.

As shown in Figure 2, a progressive reduction of the baseline nociceptive threshold was observed using a foot-withdrawal test in rats receiving repeated intrathecal morphine administration over a seven-day period (2–4). The reduced baseline nociceptive threshold was also observed in animals receiving subcutaneous fentanyl boluses using the Randall–Sellitto test in which a constantly increasing pressure is applied to a rat's hind paw (5,6). The decreased baseline nociceptive threshold lasted five days after the cessation of four fentanyl bolus injections (5). Moreover, the reduced baseline nociceptive threshold was detected in animals with repeated heroin administration (5). These results indicate that repeated opioid administration leads to a progressive and lasting reduction of the baseline nociceptive threshold, which is referred to as opioid-induced hyperalgesia.

Since hyperalgesia occurs during an opioid withdrawal, it is possible that the decreased baseline nociceptive threshold observed in these preclinical studies simply reflects a subliminal withdrawal in which changes in the baseline nociceptive threshold are present without other withdrawal signs such as wet-dog

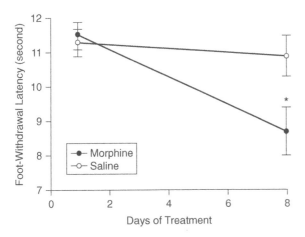

**Figure 2**  A preclinical model of opioid-induced hyperalgesia. Intrathecal administration of morphine (10 μg, once daily × 7 days) resulted in the decreased nociceptive threshold in rats as detected using a foot-withdrawal test. $*p < 0.05$, as compared with the saline group.

shake and jumping. However, a progressive reduction of the baseline nociceptive threshold is also present in animals receiving a course of continuous intrathecal opioid infusion via osmotic pumps (3,4,7). Collectively, these data support the notion that a prolonged opioid treatment not only results in the loss of the opioid antinociceptive effect, a negative sign of system adaptation (desensitization), but also leads to activation of a pronociceptive system manifested as the reduction of the nociceptive threshold, a positive sign of system adaptation (sensitization).

## NEURAL AND CELLULAR MECHANISMS UNDERLYING OPIOID-INDUCED HYPERALGESIA

If the primary effect of opioids is inhibitory at various sites of the nociceptive pathways, how would chronic opioid exposure lead to the sensitization of the central nervous system? Both opioid tolerance and opioid-induced hyperalgesia are initiated by opioid administration. It would be difficult to differentiate between these two outcomes of opioid-induced changes, if the assessment end point is a shift of opioid antinociceptive dose response curves in animal studies or a change in opioid dose demand in clinical settings. However, these two outcomes would involve two opposing cellular mechanisms, that is, a desensitization process versus a sensitization process. Because of the involvement of two opposing cellular processes, clinical approaches to resolving opioid tolerance and hyperalgesia should be different. In this regard, it is important to understand the possible neural and cellular mechanisms underlying the development of opioid-induced hyperalgesia and their interaction with the mechanism of opioid tolerance. To date, several possibilities have been raised with regard to the mechanisms of opioid-induced hyperalgesia, as briefly summarized in the following sections.

### Role of Spinal Dynorphin

It has indicated that spinal dynorphin plays an important role in the expression of both opioid tolerance and abnormal pain sensitivity (for review see Ref. 8). Of significance to note is that spinal dynorphin content increases following a period of continuous infusion with a μ-opioid receptor agonist (7). Moreover, there is an increase in the evoked release of spinal excitatory neuropeptides such as calcitonin gene-related peptide from primary afferents in morphine-treated animals, which requires the spinal dynorphin activity (9). These observations lend support to the concept that opioid administration induces a pronociceptive process, in part, by increasing the synthesis of excitatory neuropeptides and facilitating their release upon peripheral stimulation.

### Role of Descending Facilitation

Additional evidence for the involvement of a sensitization process following opioid administration comes from a group of studies that indicate the influence of descending facilitation on opioid-induced pain sensitivity. First, subsets of neurons (on- and off-cells) within the rostral ventromedial medulla (RVM) have characteristic response patterns to opioids (10,11). Their activities may contribute to the mechanisms of descending facilitation that influences spinal nociceptive processing (12). Second, on-cell activity within the RVM increases in association with the behavioral manifestation of naloxone-precipitated hyperalgesia (13). Third, bilateral lesioning of the dorsolateral funiculus, an anatomic pathway connecting the brainstem and spinal cord, blocks the increase in spinal excitatory neuropeptides in opioid-treated animals (9), suggesting that the descending facilitation may function in part through the modulation of spinal neuropeptide contents.

## Role of the Central Glutamatergic System

Activation of excitatory amino acid receptors such as the *N*-methyl-D-aspartate receptor (NMDAR) has been implicated in the mechanisms of pharmacological opioid tolerance (14,15). Subsequently, the NMDAR has been shown to be critical to the cellular mechanisms of opioid-induced hyperalgesia (2,6). The current data suggests that opioid-induced desensitization (pharmacological tolerance) and sensitization (opioid-induced hyperalgesia) processes may have many common cellular elements that are linked to the activation of the glutamatergic system.

First, inhibition of NMDAR prevents the development of both pharmacological tolerance and opioid-induced hyperalgesia (2,14,15). Second, perturbation of spinal glutamate transporter activity, which regulates extracellular glutamate availability, modulates the development of both morphine tolerance and the associated pain sensitivity (3). Third, the $Ca^{2+}$-regulated intracellular protein kinase C (PKC) is likely to be an intracellular link between cellular mechanisms of tolerance and opioid-induced hyperalgesia (2,16,17). Fourth, cross talk between the neural mechanisms of opioid tolerance and pathological pain may exist and contribute to the exacerbated pain and reduced opioid analgesic efficacy under such circumstances (18,19). Fifth, prolonged morphine administration induces NMDAR-mediated neurotoxicity in the form of apoptotic cell death, which is, at least in part, contributory to both morphine tolerance and abnormal pain sensitivity (4). Taken together, these lines of evidence strongly indicate a critical role of the central glutamatergic system in the neural mechanisms of both opioid tolerance and opioid-induced hyperalgesia.

## A Schematic Illustration of NMDAR-Mediated Cellular Mechanisms

If NMDAR were critically contributory to opioid-induced hyperalgesia, how would chronic opioid exposure result in the activation of NMDAR? Figure 3 shows the interaction between opioid receptors and NMDAR at the cellular level within the spinal cord dorsal horn, which includes a presynaptic site of primary

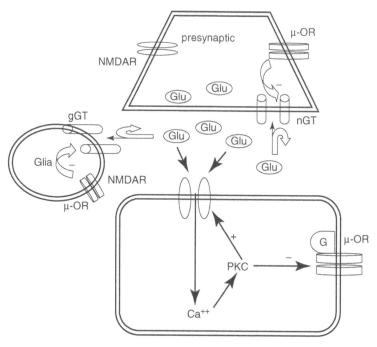

**Figure 3** Schematic illustration of the NMDAR-mediated cellular mechanisms of opioid-induced hyperalgesia (see the main text for a detailed discussion). *Abbreviations*: gGT, glial glutamate transporter; nGT, neuronal glutamate transporter; Glu, glutamate; G, G-protein; NMDAR, *N*-methyl-D-aspartate receptorl; PKC, protein kinase C.

nociceptive afferents, a postsynaptic site of projection neurons (neurons that send ascending axons to the brain) or interneurons (neurons that participate in local connections), and glial cells.

Opioid receptors (e.g., μ-opioid receptors) are present, so are NMDARs, at the presynaptic site, postsynaptic site, and glial cells. The NMDAR is a unique receptor-$Ca^{2+}$ channel complex. The activation of NMDAR leads to the opening of the $Ca^{2+}$ channel. Seated deeply inside the channel is the $Mg^{2+}$ block that is normally removed through partial depolarization of the cell membrane. This partial depolarization takes place through activation of other coexisting receptors such as non-NMDA glutamate receptors and neurokinin receptors (e.g., NK-1).

Since the predominant effect of opioid analgesics is the cell membrane hyperpolarization, which is opposite to the cell membrane excitation (cell depolarization), it would be difficult to envision that the deeply seated $Mg^{2+}$ block inside the NMDAR-$Ca^{2+}$ channel complex could be removed in the presence of the inhibitory effect of opioid analgesics. In this regard, the intra-cellular PKC plays a pivotal role in removing the $Mg^{2+}$ block in the absence of partial depolarization of the cell membrane, because chronic opioid exposure increases the PKC expression (18,19). That is, the NMDAR can be primed by

PKC activation, which is in turn induced by chronic opioid exposure. PKC activation also plays a role in the desensitization of opioid receptors. Priming NMDAR contributes to the mechanisms of opioid-induced hyperalgesia, whereas desensitizing opioid receptors contributes to the mechanisms of opioid tolerance. Moreover, chronic opioid exposure also downregulates both neuronal and glial glutamate transporters and increases the glutamate (the endogenous ligand of the NMDAR) availability at the synaptic site, further enhancing the NMDAR function. As an example of possible cellular mechanisms of opioid-induced hyperalgesia, the opioid receptor-NMDAR interaction supports the notion that chronic opioid exposure could lead to a central state of pronociceptive process. Accordingly, inhibition of NMDAR or PKC has been shown to prevent the development of opioid-induced hyperalgesia in several preclinical studies (2).

## SUMMARY

Several lines of evidence strongly support an active pronociceptive process within the central nervous system initiated by chronic opioid exposure. It is possible that the involvement of each of these cellular elements discussed in the preceding text may depend on the route (intrathecal vs. systemic) and the duration of opioid administration. For instance, the difference between the involvement of the central glutamatergic system and dynorphin is that opioid tolerance could be reduced acutely by a dynorphin antiserum but not by an NMDAR antagonist (2,7,14), although both systems are involved in the mechanisms of opioid-induced hyperalgesia. Another interesting issue is that since the descending facilitation is triggered by activation of opioid receptors, the development of opioid tolerance (a desensitization process) at the cellular level may, over time, diminish the impact of the descending facilitation on the maintenance of opioid-induced hyperalgesia.

Clinical features of opioid-induced hyperalgesia will be thoroughly discussed in other chapters. In the final chapter of this book, a detailed discussion on the clinical implications of opioid-induced hyperalgesia will be provided as well.

## REFERENCES

1. Hargreaves K, Dubner R, Brown F, et al. A new and sensitive method for measuring thermal nociception in cutaneous hyperalgesia. Pain 1988; 32:77–88.
2. Mao J, Price DD, Mayer DJ. Thermal hyperalgesia in association with the development of morphine tolerance in rats: roles of excitatory amino acid receptors and protein kinase C. J Neurosci 1994; 14:2301–2312.
3. Mao J, Sung B, Ji RR, et al. Chronic morphine induces downregulation of spinal glutamate transporters: implications in morphine tolerance and abnormal pain sensitivity. J Neurosci 2002; 22:8312–8323.
4. Mao J, Sung B, Ji RR, et al. Neuronal apoptosis associated with morphine tolerance: evidence for an opioid-induced neurotoxic mechanism. J Neurosci 2002; 22:7650–7661.

5. Celerier E, Rivat C, Jun Y, et al. Long-lasting hyperalgesia induced by fentanyl in rats: preventive effect of ketamine. Anesthesiology 2000; 92:465–472.

6. Laulin JP, Maurette P, Corcuff JB, et al. The role of ketamine in preventing fentanyl-induced hyperalgesia and subsequent acute morphine tolerance. AnesthAnalg 2002; 94:1263–1269.

7. Vanderah TW, Gardell LR, Burgess SE, et al. Dynorphin promotes abnormal pain and spinal opioid antinociceptive tolerance. J Neurosci 2000; 20:7074–7079.

8. Vanderah TW, Ossipov MH, Lai J, et al. Mechanisms of opioid-induced pain and antinociceptive tolerance: descending facilitation and spinal dynorphin. Pain 2001; 92:5–9.

9. Gardell LR, Wang R, Burgess SE, et al. Sustained morphine exposure induces a spinal dynorphin-dependent enhancement of excitatory transmitter release from primary afferent fibers. J Neurosci 2002; 22:6747–6755.

10. Barbaro NM, Heinricher MM, Fields HL. Putative pain modulating neurons in the rostral ventral medulla: reflex-related activity predicts effects of morphine. Brain Res 1986; 366:203–210.

11. Heinricher MM, Morgan MM, Fields HL. Direct and indirect actions of morphine on medullary neurons that modulate nociception. Neuroscience 1992; 48:533–543.

12. Morgan MM, Heinricher MM, Fields HL. Circuitry linking opioid-sensitive nociceptive modulatory systems in periaqueductal gray and spinal cord with rostral ventromedial medulla. Neuroscience 1992; 47:863–871.

13. Bederson JB, Fields HL, Barbaro NM. Hyperalgesia during naloxone-precipitated withdrawal from morphine is associated with increased on-cell activity in the rostral ventromedial medulla. Somatosens Mot Res 1990; 7:185–203.

14. Trujillo KA, Akil H. Inhibition of morphine tolerance and dependence by the NMDA receptor antagonist MK-801. Science 1991; 251:85–87.

15. Marek P, Ben Eliyahu S, Gold M, et al. Excitatroy amino acid antagonists (kynurenic acid and MK-801) attenuate the development of morphine tolerance in the rat. Brain Res 1991; 547:77–81.

16. Narita M, Mizoguchi H, Nagase H, et al. Involvement of spinal protein kinase Cgamma in the attenuation of opioid-μ-receptor-mediated G-protein activity after chronic intrathecal administration of [D-Ala2,N-Mephe4,Gly-Ol5]enkephalin. J Neurosci 2001; 21:3715–3720.

17. Zeitz KP, Malmberg AB, Gilbert H, et al. Reduced development of tolerance to the analgesic effects of morphine and clonidine in PKCgamma mutant mice. Pain 2002; 94:245–253.

18. Mao J, Price DD, Mayer DJ. Experimental mononeuropathy reduces the antinociceptive effects of morphine: implications for common intracellular mechanisms involved in morphine tolerance and neuropathic pain. Pain 1995; 61:353–364.

19. Mao J. NMDA and opioid receptors: their interactions in antinociception, tolerance and neuroplasticity. Brain Res Rev 1999; 30:289–304.

# 2

# Cellular Mechanisms Underlying Morphine Analgesic Tolerance and Hyperalgesia

**Hiroshi Ueda**

*Division of Molecular Pharmacology and Neuroscience, Graduate School of Biomedical Sciences, Nagasaki University, Nagasaki, Japan*

## INTRODUCTION

Opioid dose escalation or analgesic tolerance is observed during longer treatments in a significant number of patients with chronic pain owing to cancer or nonmalignant tissue injury. Higher doses of morphine are more likely to result in subsensitivity to the drug and worsened quality of life (QOL) by exerting other side effects. Many investigators have been studying the molecular and cellular mechanisms underlying opioid analgesic tolerance by different approaches. They studied the underlying mechanisms in terms of cellular opioid adaptation following long-term exposure. In so-called cyclic AMP hypothesis in mid-1970s, adapted loss of opioid-mediated inhibition of cyclic AMP production and abrupt increase in this level following opioid withdrawal were proposed as mechanistic models for opioid tolerance and dependence, respectively (1–3). In the current cellular models, it is well documented that the molecular events underlying the reduction of opioid receptor function following morphine pre-treatments are closely correlated with receptor trafficking, including (*i*) phosphorylation, (*ii*) internalization/endocytosis, (*iii*) sequestration/recycling, or (*iv*) downregulation/breakdown of these receptors (4–8). Among these steps, the phosphorylation of opioid receptors is the most important step for desensitization. The direct evidence that opioid receptor function is lost by phosphorylation has been first reported in the studies using partially purified μ-opioid receptors (MOPs) and purified cAMP-dependent protein kinase (PKA) (9–11). It is accepted that longer exposure to opioids leads to phosphorylation of the C-terminal region of opioid receptors, followed by desensitization (12,13). However, there are reports that opioid receptors are phosphorylated by many different kinases, and details of the proposed opioid receptor phosphorylation and trafficking machineries underlying opioid tolerance and desensitization have been described elsewhere (9,14–21).

In addition to these cellular mechanisms, the plasticity in neuronal counterbalancing mechanisms including different neurons has also been proposed as a possible mechanism underlying opioid tolerance. The rationality of this plasticity is found in the fact that the degree of tolerance differs in different opioid actions. The morphine-induced respiratory inhibition and analgesia is known to develop tolerance, while the constipation is not (22–25). Trujillo and Akil (1991) first reported that MK-801, an *N*-methyl-D-aspartic acid (NMDA) receptor antagonist, blocks opioid tolerance and dependence (26). This finding suggests that the anti-opioid NMDA receptor system is enhanced during chronic opioid treatments, thereby counteracting the actions of opioids. This type of plasticity through anti-opioid NMDA receptor system seems to be augmented by various supporting mechanisms, as described later.

## PLASTICITY IN NEURONAL NETWORKS

The plasticity in central neuronal networks underlying the mechanism of opioid tolerance following chronic treatments may be evidenced by the following study (27,28). Although the morphine analgesia assessed by the tail pinch test, which involves higher central nervous mechanisms, was markedly attenuated on the sixth day following daily systemic injection of morphine at a relatively high dose of 10 mg/kg (SC), the peripheral morphine analgesia was not observed in such morphine-tolerant mice. In this study, the peripheral morphine analgesia by local (intraplantar, IPl) injection was evaluated to measure the inhibition of nociceptive flexor responses by bradykinin (IPl). Thus the discrepancy in susceptibility to chronic morphine analgesic tolerance seems to be attributed to the absence (peripheral) or presence of neuronal circuits (systemic or central) that affect morphine analgesia. Most importantly, the tolerance to peripheral morphine analgesia was not observed as late as 24 hours later. Therefore, we must separately consider the molecular mechanisms underlying acute and chronic morphine analgesic tolerance in terms of synaptic plasticity. Although accumulated findings demonstrate that several brain loci are closely related to the cause of morphine analgesia (29), it remains unclear whether the neuronal plasticity involved in morphine analgesic tolerance is caused by locus-specific or translocus systems.

## Anti-Opioid Glutamate-NMDA Receptor System

Since the report by Trujillo and Akil (1991), NMDA receptors have long been supposed to play important roles in the development of morphine tolerance and dependence (30,31). As many known competitive or noncompetitive NMDA antagonists potentiate morphine-induced catalepsy, lethality (32), and hypo-thermia (33), or retard learning behaviors (34), the development of NMDA receptor antagonists that specifically block morphine tolerance has been explored. One approach to find specific antagonists began with the identification of the subunit of NMDA receptor involved in morphine tolerance and addiction. We first revealed that GluRepsilon1 (NR2A) knockout mice showed an enhancement of acute morphine analgesia in the tail pinch test (35). As NR2A knockout mice did not show any change in the basal nociceptive threshold, glutamatergic neurons that stimulate NR2A subunit are located downstream of opioid neurons, and attenuate endogenous and exogenous opioid actions. Chronic daily pretreatments with morphine (10 mg/kg SC) produced a tolerance to morphine analgesia on the 6th day in wild-type mice, but not in NR2A knockout mice. As the level of NR2A was significantly increased by 100 to 200% of the control level only in the periaqueductal gray matter (PAG), ventral tegmental area (VTA), and nucleus accumbens (NAcc), we speculated that enhanced activation of the anti-opioid NMDA receptor system counterbalances or cancels morphine analgesia during chronic treatments. The restoration of this gene through a novel in vivo electroporation technique into the PAG or VTA, but not the NAcc of NR2A knockout mice, successfully restored the morphine analgesic tolerance, without significant changes in the basal nociceptive threshold (Fig. 1). The rescued NR2A protein level by in vivo electroporation (1 μg DNA, 10 mA and 10 Hz) in the PAG was almost the same as that in wild-type mice, and remained at this level until nine days after electroporation, although the nonspecific CMV promoter is used for NR2A gene transfer. It probably suggests that extra-NR2A proteins not used for the right NMDA receptor complex may be removed by protein quality-check systems, such as ubiquitin-proteasome system (36).

Our developed technique also has the advantage that it caused no mor-phological damage to the PAG under the condition with 10 to 40 mA at 10 Hz, or with 10 and 20 Hz at 10 mA at day 4 after in vivo electroporation, although slightly fragmented nuclei were observed with 40 Hz at 10 mA. Similar approaches were carried out to study the mechanisms underlying morphine dependence. Mice given increasing doses of morphine from 20 to 100 mg/kg for three days showed withdrawal behaviors when 1 mg/kg IP naloxone was administered two hours after the last morphine (100 mg/kg SC) injection on the fourth day. The withdrawal behaviors such as jumping, withdrawal locomotion,

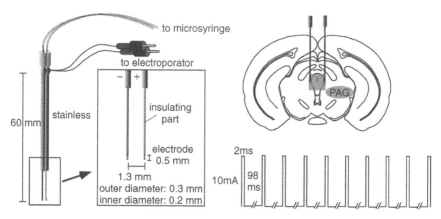

**Figure 1** Method for in vivo electroporation. A pair of stainless steel electrodes, 0.5 mm in length and 0.3 mm in outer diameter, was stereotaxically inserted into specific brain regions according to the stereotaxic atlas in anesthetized mice. Electric pulses were generated with a square electroporator (CUY21, Nepagene, Tokyo, Japan) at 10 pulses/s (10 Hz). The shape of the pulse was a square wave; that is, the voltage remained constant during the pulse duration. For the best gene transfer, cDNA at a dose of 1 μg was diluted in Tris-EDTA buffer (1 μL) immediately before use and electroporated into brain regions by the electric pulses (2 ms) to get 10 mA current.

sniffing, and defecation were similarly observed by both paradigms of morphine treatments. These withdrawal behaviors were markedly inhibited in NR2A knockout mice and there was a significant increase in protein expression of NR2A of wild-type mice. Locus-specific recovery of some, but not all withdrawal behaviors was observed when NR2A gene expression was restored in the NAcc of knockout mice, suggesting that both locus-specific and translocus NR2A systems are involved in the development of opioid dependence. Thus, we propose the view that enhanced anti-opioid systems may attenuate the actions of morphine following chronic morphine treatments, and deprivation from morphine may lead to withdrawal symptoms through anti-opioid NR2A systems.

On the other hand, NR2B has also been proposed to contribute to the mechanisms of morphine tolerance or the plasticity in opioid actions. Ro 256981, an antagonist of the NMDA receptor subunit NR2B, reduces the expression of analgesic tolerance to morphine (37). Since NMDA NR2B receptors in the anterior cingulated cortex (ACC) play roles in the establishment of long-term potentiation (LTP) and fear memory, both systemic and intra-ACC inhibition of NR2B in morphine-tolerant animals inhibited the expression of analgesic tolerance. Although there is an abundance of evidence from animal studies that NMDA receptor inhibition using antagonists during opioid exposure attenuates chronic opioid tolerance, there are also some reports that NMDA receptor antagonists potentiate, inhibit, or do not alter morphine analgesia, possibly due to the use of different doses of antagonist and morphine, as well as experimental animals and tests for nociception (38). In addition, there are reports that different types of glutamate receptors are also involved in the development of opioid analgesic tolerance. Kozela et al. (2003) have pointed out the role of metabotropic glutamate receptor 5 (mGluR5) by showing that chronic administration of 2-methyl-6-(phenylethynyl)-pyridine (MPEP), a specific antagonist of group 1 mGluRs, markedly attenuated morphine tolerance (39).

## Intracellular Systems That Support The Anti-Opioid NMDA Receptor System

The knockdown of spinal cord postsynaptic density protein-95 (PSD-95), a scaffold protein for NMDA receptors, prevented the development of morphine tolerance in rats (40). On the other hand, microarray studies revealed increased expression of Ania-3, a short variant of Homer 1 protein, in the frontal cortices of rats showing naloxone-precipitated morphine withdrawal (41). As Ania-3 interferes with the function of constitutively active long forms of Homer proteins, which build bridges between NMDA and metabotropic glutamate receptors (42), this change in Ania-3 expression may contribute to the development of morphine dependence, or tolerance. These findings are consistent with the recent studies (43), in which chronic morphine upregulates the gene expression of PSD-95 and Homer-1 in the central extended amygdala, a key site for the drug craving and seeking behaviors. On the other hand, there is a report that cyclin-dependent kinase 5 (Cdk5) levels were markedly reduced in the prefrontal cortices of opioid addicts and the cerebral cortices of morphine-sensitized rats (44). These findings seem to be very interesting, since Cdk5 phosphorylates the NR2A subunit and activates NMDA receptor function (45), while the inhibition of Cdk5 increases Src-mediated phosphorylation of NR2B and blocks the binding to AP-2, resulting in the promotion of cell surface expression of NMDA receptors (46). However, there is a conflicting report that no significant change in Cdk5 expression was observed in similar brain regions of morphine-sensitized rats (43).

## BDNF System That Supports Anti-Opioid NMDA Receptor Systems

Although NR2A receptor upregulation following chronic morphine treatments seems to play a key role in the above-mentioned hypothesized mechanisms, details of mechanisms underlying NR2A upregulation remain to be determined. We speculate from the recent findings that brain-derived neurotrophic factor (BDNF) may support this anti-opioid system as follows: (*i*) the addition of BDNF to cultured rat cortical neurons upregulates NR2A gene expression (47), (*ii*) morphine upregulates BDNF expression in cultured microglia through an autocrine machinery (48), (*iii*) chronic morphine treatments upregulate BDNF expression in brain neurons in vivo through a neuron-microglia interaction (49), (*iv*) central injection of anti-BDNF antibody abolished morphine tolerance (50), and (*v*) morphine physical dependence was lost in forebrain-specific BDNF knockout mice (51). Although little is known about the molecular mechanisms underlying BDNF-induced NR2A gene expression, three functional GC-boxes in the NR2A core promoter are reported to interact with Sp1 and Sp4 transcription factors. It is interesting to speculate that the phosphorylation signaling through BDNF-TrkB couples with the transcriptional activity of Sp1 (52,53).

On the other hand, the machinery underlying chronic morphine-induced upregulation of BDNF expression is also an interesting subject. When mice were pretreated with morphine at a dose of 10 mg/kg SC (a maximal dose for analgesia) for five days, the substantial analgesic activity of morphine (10 mg/kg, SC) was lost on the 6th day. At this time point, there was a significant upregulation of BDNF levels in the PAG (50), which is the major brain region involved in morphine analgesia. However, these results seem to conflict with a report that forebrain-specific BDNF knockout mice lose morphine physical dependence, but not morphine analgesic tolerance (51). This contradictory observation is unlikely to be important because it is well known that lower brain stem regions, but not forebrain regions, are important for morphine analgesia. Indeed, the injection of adenovirus expressing Cre recombinase gene into the PAG of floxed BDNF-transgenic mice markedly reduced morphine analgesic tolerance (Matsushita and Ueda, unpublished data). We recently found that curcumin, an inhibitor of histone acetyltransferase (HAT) activity of CREB-binding protein inhibitor, blocked the chronic morphine-induced expression of exon I and IV BDNF transcripts, and morphine analgesic tolerance (50). As CBP is known to cause a chromatin remodeling through HAT activity and stimulate BDNF gene expression, these findings may be the first evidence that morphine analgesia could be suppressed by epigenetic regulation. This also indicates that a health food product, curcumin, might reduce morphine analgesic tolerance, and that underlying epigenetic control could be a new strategy useful for the control of this problem.

### Glial Systems That Support Anti-Opioid NMDA Receptor Systems

Astrocytes play important roles in the anti-opioid glutamate-NMDA receptor system. As the expression levels of glutamate transporters in astrocytes and neurons are downregulated by chronic morphine treatments (30,54), glutamate signals in the synaptic cleft are expected to increase and give more opportunity for the stimulation of NMDA receptors. On the other hand, D-serine, a key molecule that activates NMDA receptors as an allosteric agonist (55), is also a candidate of supporting machineries involved in this anti-opioid system, since chronic morphine induced the upregulation of glial racemase, which is expected to increase D-serine levels (56). Glial cell responses to chronic morphine treatment were examined by immunohistochemistry of glial fibrillary acidic protein (GFAP), a specific marker for astroglial cells (57). Chronic administration of morphine (50 mg/kg, IP, once daily for nine consecutive days) increased the immunoreactive level of GFAP, a specific marker for astroglial cells, in the spinal cord, posterior cingulate cortex, and hippocampus, but not in the thalamus. This increase was attributed primarily to hypertrophy of astroglial cells rather than their proliferation or migration. When chronic morphine (20 μg/2 μL, IT) was delivered in combination with fluorocitrate (1 nmol/L μL, IT), a specific and reversible inhibitor of glial cells, spinal tolerance to morphine analgesia was partly but significantly attenuated as measured by behavioral tests and the increase in spinal GFAP immunostaining was also greatly blocked. This report may be the first evidence for the role of glial cells in the development of morphine tolerance in vivo.

On the other hand, accumulating findings demonstrate that microglia also play key roles in morphine actions or analgesic tolerance. Takayama and Ueda (2005) reported that morphine upregulates microglial gene expression of BDNF, which is known to upregulate NR2A. However, the BDNF-like immunoreactivity in the brains of chronic morphine-treated mice was mostly observed in neurons, but slightly in microglia (Ueda et al., unpublished data). This selective expression is very intriguing because morphine upregulates BDNF expression in cultured microglia, but not in cultured neurons. From this point of view, we are attempting to find microglia-derived bioactive molecules, which in turn upregulate BDNF in neurons, followed by the development of tolerance via an upregulation of NR2A, as mentioned earlier. Liu et al. have recently reported that a selective nNOS inhibitor, 7-nitroindazole (7-NINA, sodium salt), attenuated morphine analgesic tolerance and p38 MAPK in the activated spinal microglia (58). Taking into consideration that NMDA receptor mediates an activation of nNOS, it is interesting to speculate that microglia activation downstream of NMDA receptor activation may exert an amplifying mechanism for the anti-opioid NMDA receptor systems.

## CONCLUSION

Opioids are becoming more widely used, not only as palliative medicines for terminal cancer patients, but also as successful analgesics for neuropathic pain patients. When the side effects such as tolerance and dependence are appropriately avoided by the use of adjuvant analgesics, which will be developed through the studies of underlying mechanisms, the pain control by opioids will be more idealistic. The present review proposes several target analgesic adjuvants for use in palliative care (Fig. 2). They are NR2A-specific antagonists and compounds that suppress BDNF transcription, such as curcumin. Various types of compounds to inhibit the activation of microglia, astrocytes, racemase, and nNOS would be also added to the lineup of adjuvants to inhibit opioid analgesic tolerance.

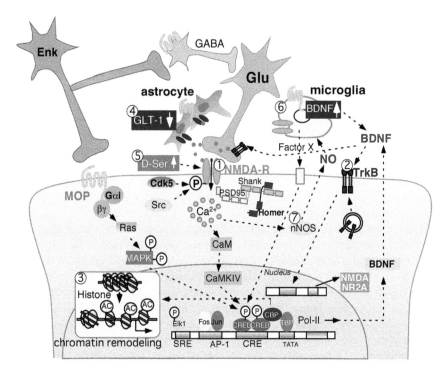

**Figure 2** Candidate molecules to inhibit opioid tolerance in the anti-opioid glutamate/ NMDA receptor hypothesis. In this hypothesis, glutamate neurotransmission and NMDA receptor signaling are upregulated, following chronic opioid treatments. Some parts of this hypothesized mechanism are mediated by neuron-glia interactions, as stated in the text. Candidate molecules to inhibit opioid tolerance are indicated by the number in the figure, as follows: (*i*) NMDA receptor (NR2A) antagonists; (*ii*) anti-BDNF antibody or TrkB antagonists; (*iii*) CBP inhibitors, such as curcumin; (*iv*) unknown compounds to inhibit the GLT-1 downregulation, racemase inhibitors; (*v*) astrocyte inactivators, such as fluorocitrate; (*vi*) microglia inactivators, such as minocycline; and (*vii*) nNOS inhibitors.

## ACKNOWLEDGMENTS

Parts of this study were supported by grants-in-aid for Scientific Research (S) (to H.U., 17109015), on Priority Areas—Research on Pathomechanisms of Brain Disorders (to H.U., 17025031, 18023028, 20023022) from the Ministry of Education, Culture, Sports, Science and Technology (MEXT).

## REFERENCES

1. Brandt M, Fischer K, Moroder L, et al. Enkephalin evokes biochemical correlates of opiate tolerance and dependence in neuroblastoma x glioma hybrid cells. FEBS Lett 1976; 68(1):38–40.

2. Collier HO, Francis DL. Morphine abstinence is associated with increased brain cyclic AMP. Nature 1975; 255(5504):159–162.
3. Sharma SK, Klee WA, Nirenberg M. Dual regulation of adenylate cyclase accounts for narcotic dependence and tolerance. Proc Natl Acad Sci U S A 1975; 72(8): 3092–3096.
4. Christie MJ. Cellular neuroadaptations to chronic opioids: tolerance, withdrawal and addiction. Br J Pharmacol 2008; 154(2):384–396.
5. Koch T, Hollt V. Role of receptor internalization in opioid tolerance and dependence. Pharmacol Ther 2008; 117(2):199–206.
6. Marie N, Aguila B, Allouche S. Tracking the opioid receptors on the way of desensitization. Cell Signal 2006; 18(11):1815–1833.
7. Martini L, Whistler JL. The role of mu opioid receptor desensitization and endocytosis in morphine tolerance and dependence. Curr Opin Neurobiol 2007; 17(5): 556–564.
8. Wang ZJ, Wang LX. Phosphorylation: a molecular switch in opioid tolerance. Life Sci 2006; 79(18):1681–1691.
9. Harada H, Ueda H, Katada T, et al. Phosphorylated mu-opioid receptor purified from rat brains lacks functional coupling with Gi1, a GTP-binding protein in reconstituted lipid vesicles. Neurosci Lett 1990; 113(1):47–49.
10. Harada H, Ueda H, Wada Y, et al. Phosphorylation of mu-opioid receptors—a putative mechanism of selective uncoupling of receptor—Gi interaction, measured with low-Km GTPase and nucleotide-sensitive agonist binding. Neurosci Lett 1989; 100(1–3):221–226.
11. Ueda H, Harada H, Nozaki M, et al. Reconstitution of rat brain mu opioid receptors with purified guanine nucleotide-binding regulatory proteins, Gi and Go. Proc Natl Acad Sci USA 1988; 85(18):7013–7017.
12. Afify EA, Law PY, Riedl M, et al. Role of carboxyl terminus of mu-and delta-opioid receptor in agonist-induced down-regulation. Brain Res Mol Brain Res 1998; 54(1): 24–34.
13. Pak Y, O'Dowd BF, George SR. Agonist-induced desensitization of the mu opioid receptor is determined by threonine 394 preceded by acidic amino acids in the COOH-terminal tail. J Biol Chem 1997; 272(40):24961–24965.
14. Belcheva MM, Szucs M, Wang D, et al. mu-Opioid receptor-mediated ERK activation involves calmodulin-dependent epidermal growth factor receptor transactivation. J Biol Chem 2001; 276(36):33847–33853.
15. Gucker S, Bidlack JM. Protein kinase C activation increases the rate and magnitude of agonist-induced delta-opioid receptor down-regulation in NG108-15 cells. Mol Pharmacol 1992; 42(4):656–665.
16. Koch T, Kroslak T, Mayer P, et al. Site mutation in the rat mu-opioid receptor demonstrates the involvement of calcium/calmodulin-dependent protein kinase II in agonist-mediated desensitization. J Neurochem 1997; 69(4):1767–1770.
17. Pei G, Kieffer BL, Lefkowitz RJ, et al. Agonist-dependent phosphorylation of the mouse delta-opioid receptor: involvement of G protein-coupled receptor kinases but not protein kinase C. Mol Pharmacol 1995; 48(2):173–177.
18. Polakiewicz RD, Schieferl SM, Dorner LF, et al. A mitogen-activated protein kinase pathway is required for μ-opioid receptor desensitization. J Biol Chem 1998; 273(20): 12402–12406.

19. Ueda H, Miyamae T, Hayashi C, et al. Protein kinase C involvement in homologous desensitization of delta-opioid receptor coupled to Gi1-phospholipase C activation in Xenopus oocytes. J Neurosci 1995; 15(11):7485–7499.

20. Ueda H, Ueda M. Mechanisms underlying morphine analgesic tolerance and dependence—involvements of protein kinase C and anti-opioid glutamate-NMDA receptor system. Frontiers in Bioscience—regulation and function of opioid receptor genes. 2009; 14:5260–5272.

21. Zhang J, Ferguson SS, Barak LS, et al. Role for G protein-coupled receptor kinase in agonist-specific regulation of mu-opioid receptor responsiveness. Proc Natl Acad Sci USA 1998; 95(12):7157–7162.

22. Ling GS, Paul D, Simantov R, et al. Differential development of acute tolerance to analgesia, respiratory depression, gastrointestinal transit and hormone release in a morphine infusion model. Life Sci 1989; 45(18):1627–1636.

23. Thompson AR, Ray JB. The importance of opioid tolerance: a therapeutic paradox. J Am Coll Surg 2003; 196(2):321–324.

24. Yuan CS, Foss JF, O'Connor M, et al. Gut motility and transit changes in patients receiving long-term methadone maintenance. J Clin Pharmacol 1998; 38(10):931–935.

25. Gutstein HB, Akil H. Opioid analgesics. In: Bunton LL, Lazo JS, Parker KL, eds. Goodman & Gilman's The Pharmacological Basis of Therapeutics. 11th ed. New York, NY: McGraw-Hill; 2006:547–590.

26. Trujillo KA, Akil H. Inhibition of morphine tolerance and dependence by the NMDA receptor antagonist MK-801. Science 1991; 251(4989):85–87.

27. Ueda H, Inoue M. Peripheral morphine analgesia resistant to tolerance in chronic morphine-treated mice. Neurosci Lett 1999; 266(2):105–108.

28. Ueda H, Inoue M, Matsumoto T. Protein kinase C-mediated inhibition of mu-opioid receptor internalization and its involvement in the development of acute tolerance to peripheral mu-agonist analgesia. J Neurosci 2001; 21(9):2967–2973.

29. Manning BH, Morgan MJ, Franklin KB. Morphine analgesia in the formalin test: evidence for forebrain and midbrain sites of action. Neuroscience 1994; 63(1):289–294.

30. Mao J, Sung B, Ji RR, et al. Chronic morphine induces downregulation of spinal glutamate transporters: implications in morphine tolerance and abnormal pain sensitivity. J Neurosci 2002; 22(18):8312–8323.

31. Trujillo KA. Are NMDA receptors involved in opiate-induced neural and behavioral plasticity? A review of preclinical studies. Psychopharmacology (Berlin) 2000; 151 (2-3):121–141.

32. Trujillo KA, Akil H. The NMDA receptor antagonist MK-801 increases morphine catalepsy and lethality. Pharmacol Biochem Behav 1991; 38(3):673–675.

33. Bhargava HN. Enhancement of morphine actions in morphine-naive and morphine-tolerant mice by LY 235959, a competitive antagonist of the NMDA receptor. Gen Pharmacol 1997; 28(1):61–64.

34. Bannerman DM, Rawlins JN, Good MA. The drugs don't work-or do they? Pharmacological and transgenic studies of the contribution of NMDA and GluR-A-containing AMPA receptors to hippocampal-dependent memory. Psychopharmacology (Berlin) 2006; 188(4):552–566.

35. Inoue M, Mishina M, Ueda H. Locus-specific rescue of GluRepsilon1 NMDA receptors in mutant mice identifies the brain regions important for morphine tolerance and dependence. J Neurosci 2003; 23(16):6529–6536.

36. Ravid T, Hochstrasser M. Diversity of degradation signals in the ubiquitin-proteasome system. Nat Rev Mol Cell Biol 2008; 9(9):679–690.
37. Ko SW, Wu LJ, Shum F, et al. Cingulate NMDA NR2B receptors contribute to morphine-induced analgesic tolerance. Mol Brain 2008; 1(1):2.
38. Kozela E, Popik P. The effects of NMDA receptor antagonists on acute morphine antinociception in mice. Amino Acids 2002; 23(1–3):163–168.
39. Kozela E, Pilc A, Popik P. Inhibitory effects of MPEP, an mGluR5 antagonist, and memantine, an *N*-methyl-D-aspartate receptor antagonist, on morphine antinociceptive tolerance in mice. Psychopharmacology (Berlin) 2003; 165(3):245–251.
40. Liaw WJ, Zhang B, Tao F, et al. Knockdown of spinal cord postsynaptic density protein-95 prevents the development of morphine tolerance in rats. Neuroscience 2004; 123(1):11–15.
41. Ammon S, Mayer P, Riechert U, et al. Microarray analysis of genes expressed in the frontal cortex of rats chronically treated with morphine and after naloxone precipitated withdrawal. Brain Res Mol Brain Res 2003; 112(1–2):113–125.
42. Yang L, Mao L, Tang Q, et al. A novel $Ca^{2+}$-independent signaling pathway to extracellular signal-regulated protein kinase by coactivation of NMDA receptors and metabotropic glutamate receptor 5 in neurons. J Neurosci 2004; 24(48):10846–10857.
43. Befort K, Filliol D, Ghate A, et al. Mu-opioid receptor activation induces transcriptional plasticity in the central extended amygdala. Eur J Neurosci 2008; 27(11): 2973–2984.
44. Ferrer-Alcon M, La Harpe R, Guimon J, et al. Downregulation of neuronal cdk5/p35 in opioid addicts and opiate-treated rats: relation to neurofilament phosphorylation. Neuropsychopharmacology 2003; 28(5):947–955.
45. Li BS, Sun MK, Zhang L, et al. Regulation of NMDA receptors by cyclin-dependent kinase-5. Proc Natl Acad Sci U S A 2001; 98(22), 12742–12747.
46. Zhang S, Edelmann L, Liu J, et al. Cdk5 regulates the phosphorylation of tyrosine 1472 NR2B and the surface expression of NMDA receptors. J Neurosci 2008; 28(2): 415–424.
47. Small DL, Murray CL, Mealing GA, et al. Brain derived neurotrophic factor induction of *N*-methyl-D-aspartate receptor subunit NR2A expression in cultured rat cortical neurons. Neurosci Lett 1998; 252(3):211–214.
48. Takayama N, Ueda H. Morphine-induced chemotaxis and brain-derived neurotrophic factor expression in microglia. J Neurosci 2005; 25(2):430–435.
49. Yonekubo S, Matsushita Y, Ueda H. Microglia activation is involved in the initiation of morphine analgesic tolerance. INRC, Charleston, SC, 2008:46.
50. Matsushita Y, Ueda H. Curcumin blocks chronic morphine analgesic tolerance and brain-derived neurotrophic factor upregulation. Neuroreport 2009; 20(1):63–68.
51. Akbarian S, Rios M, Liu RJ, et al. Brain-derived neurotrophic factor is essential for opiate-induced plasticity of noradrenergic neurons. J Neurosci 2002; 22(10): 4153–4162.
52. Deng X, Yellaturu C, Cagen L, et al. Expression of the rat sterol regulatory element-binding protein-1c gene in response to insulin is mediated by increased transactivating capacity of specificity protein 1 (Sp1). J Biol Chem 2007; 282(24):17517–17529.
53. Solomon SS, Majumdar G, Martinez-Hernandez A, et al. A critical role of Sp1 transcription factor in regulating gene expression in response to insulin and other hormones. Life Sci 2008; 83(9–10):305–312.

54. Ozawa T, Nakagawa T, Shige K, et al. Changes in the expression of glial glutamate transporters in the rat brain accompanied with morphine dependence and naloxone-precipitated withdrawal. Brain Res 2001; 905(1–2):254–258.

55. Johnson JW, Ascher P. Glycine potentiates the NMDA response in cultured mouse brain neurons. Nature 1987; 325(6104):529–531.

56. Yoshikawa M, Shinomiya T, Takayasu N, et al. Long-term treatment with morphine increases the D-serine content in the rat brain by regulating the mRNA and protein expressions of serine racemase and D-amino acid oxidase. J Pharmacol Sci 2008; 107(3):270–276.

57. Song P, Zhao ZQ. The involvement of glial cells in the development of morphine tolerance. Neurosci Res 2001; 39(3):281–286.

58. Liu W, Wang C-H, Cui, Y, et al. Inhibition of neuronal nitric oxide synthase antagonizes morphine antinociceptive tolerance by decreasing activation of p38 MAPK in the spinal microglia. Neurosci Lett 2006; 410(3):174–177.

# 3

# Overview on Clinical Features of Opioid-Induced Hyperalgesia

**Martin S. Angst and Larry F. Chu**

*Stanford University School of Medicine, Stanford, California, U.S.A.*

**J. David Clark**

*Stanford University School of Medicine and Palo Alto Veterans Affairs Hospital, Palo Alto, California, U.S.A.*

## INTRODUCTION

A growing body of literature suggests that patients receiving opioids for pain control, somewhat paradoxically, may develop an increased sensitivity to pain as a direct consequence of that therapy (1–5). This phenomenon has been termed "opioid-induced hyperalgesia" (OIH). Thus, the clinical use of opioids may be a double-edged sword, initially offering pain relief but subsequently evoking hyperalgesia.

A large number of animal studies have documented OIH resulting from the administration of various types of opioids in models of acute and chronic pain. The number of human studies investigating OIH is significantly smaller. Most of these studies are cross-sectional in design and have compared different study populations at one time. As such, these studies do not allow rigorous inference as to the cause of observed differences and provide only indirect evidence for the development of OIH. However, a few studies used a prospective design and followed subjects over time. Data from these studies provide the best and most direct evidence for the development of OIH. In light of accumulating experimental data corroborating the view that OIH does develop in humans, it is important to note that studies elucidating the clinical significance of OIH are sparse.

The aim of this chapter is to examine existing data concerning the development of OIH in humans, discuss potential clinical implications of OIH, and identify key questions in need of an answer. Other chapters in this book will specifically focus on the clinical assessment of OIH, the impact and therapy of OIH in various clinical settings, and the connection between OIH and tolerance, dependence, and addiction.

## CLINICAL PRESENTATION

The development of OIH has been described in distinct clinical settings that are characterized by the opioid dose and the pattern of its administration: (*i*) OIH during opioid maintenance therapy and withdrawal, (*ii*) OIH when using ultra-high and escalating doses, and (iii) OIH that may occur at ultralow and sub-clinical doses (1,2). In this chapter, emphasis will be placed on OIH during opioid maintenance therapy and withdrawal. It is likely that this type of OIH is the most relevant to patient care.

## OIH During Maintenance and Withdrawal

Most studies in humans reported OIH during ongoing opioid therapy or with-drawal from opioids. In fact, pain has long been known to be associated with opioid withdrawal, and today pain is considered as one of the criteria for the diagnosis of withdrawal (6,7). However, clinical scientists only recently became interested in systematically addressing the question of whether OIH develops in humans. This interest was largely triggered by animal studies suggesting that OIH may impact the utility of opioids in pain therapy.

Evidence so far suggests that OIH does develop in humans and may have important clinical implications. Data supporting this view have been collected in five distinct settings: (*i*) in former opioid addicts maintained on methadone, (*ii*) in chronic pain patients, (*iii*) during opioid detoxification, (*iv*) in patients undergoing surgery, and (*v*) in human volunteers tested in experimental pain paradigms. Data generated in these studies will be discussed in the following paragraphs.

### Former Opioid Addicts Maintained on Methadone

Studies in former opioid addicts maintained on methadone are among the first investigations reporting evidence for the development of OIH in humans (8–14). Several clinical investigators have measured pain sensitivity in former addicts with aid of experimental pain models. Results obtained from the cold pressor test consistently suggest that former addicts maintained on an average daily meth-adone dose of 60 to 70 mg were more sensitive to pain than former addicts not maintained on methadone or healthy controls. During the cold pressure test subjects are asked to immerse their hands in ice water and the time is measured until they withdraw their hands because of intolerable pain. While differences in sensitivity to cold pressor pain were remarkable (40–80%), hardly any differences were detected when assessing sensitivity to mechanical or electrically induced pain.

Cold pressor pain differs from mechanical or electrically induced pain because it evokes a significantly stronger negative affective response to pain (15). One can hypothesize that differences in affective response to pain rather than differences in pain intensity distinguished former addicts on methadone from control groups. This view is supported by a study documenting that addicts on methadone withdrew their hands from an ice water bath at significantly lower pain intensities than subjects in control groups (16). Taken together, these results are compatible with the view that addicts maintained on methadone were more annoyed or bothered by cold pressor pain, but did not experience cold pressor pain at greater intensities than subjects in control groups. It also remains unclear whether an increased sensitivity to cold pressor pain was a consequence of opioid consumption or, alternatively, a unique characteristic of subjects vulnerable for developing addictive diseases. An increased sensitivity to cold pressor pain has also been reported in cocaine addicts (8). Thus, the validity of using "cold pressor pain sensitivity" as a marker of OIH requires backing from prospective clinical studies.

## Chronic Pain Patients on Opioid Therapy

A prospective study in a small number of patients suffering from chronic low back pain reported development of OIH, as indicated by an increased sensitivity to cold pressor pain one month after initiating oral morphine therapy (17). While prospective in character, reported findings are limited because the study did not include a control group. Several cross-sectional studies also searched for evidence of OIH in chronic pain patients by comparing pain sensitivity between opioid-treated and opioid-naive patients (18–21). Findings of these studies are summarized in Table 1. Investigators used various pain modalities to test for OIH. Evidence for the development of OIH was provided by two of three studies examining pain sensitivity with aid of the cold pressor test (17–19). Consistent with data collected in former opioid addicts on methadone maintenance, other conventional tests using heat, electrical, or mechanical stimuli to evoke pain failed to detect differences in pain sensitivity between opioid-naive and opioid-treated patients.

As discussed previously, it is of some concern that the development of OIH in chronic pain patients and former addicts on methadone maintenance is inferred almost exclusively from cold pressor pain data. In this respect, results from two recent studies using novel pain test paradigms are particularly interesting. Both studies provide evidence for the development of OIH during chronic

**Table 1** Studies in Chronic Pain Patients

| Reference | Pain | Patients | Dose[a] | Length[b] | Pain model | | | | | | |
|---|---|---|---|---|---|---|---|---|---|---|---|
| | | | | | CPP | HP | IP | MP | EP | DNIC | LA |
| Fillingim (21) | Nonmalignant (back pain) | 240 | 250 | ? | – | – | ND | – | – | – | – |
| Reznikow (20) | Nonmalignant or cancer | 224 | 70 | 9 | – | ND | – | ND | – | – | – |
| Chu (17) | Nonmalignant (back pain) | 6 | 60 | 1 | 40%↑ | ND | – | – | – | – | – |
| Hay (19) | Nonmalignant | 40 | 250 | 46 | 60%↑ | – | – | – | ND | – | – |
| Ram (18) | Nonmalignant or cancer | 110 | 100 | 20 | ND | – | – | – | – | 40%↓ | – |
| Cohen (22) | Nonmalignant or cancer | 382 | 100 | 64 | – | – | – | – | – | – | 20%↑ |

[a] Average or median daily oral morphine equivalents (mg).
[b] Duration of opioid therapy (month).
*Abbreviations:* CPP, cold pressor test; HP, heat pain; IP, ischemic pain; MP, mechanical pain; EP, electrical pain; DNIC, diffuse noxious inhibitory control; LA, pain on injection of a local anesthetic.

opioid therapy. One study measured efficiency of diffuse noxious inhibitory control (DNIC) mechanisms for suppressing pain. DNIC was significantly attenuated in pain patients on chronic opioid therapy, which could explain their increased sensitivity to pain (18). The second study examined pain when injecting a local anesthetic prior to needle insertion for an interventional procedure. Pain on injection was greater if patients were on chronic opioid therapy and directly correlated with the daily opioid dose and the duration of opioid therapy (22).

## Opioid Detoxification

Two studies formally examined OIH during opioid detoxification of chronic pain patients or opioid addicts consuming heroin and/or methadone (16,23). Both studies used the cold pressor test to quantify pain sensitivity. Sensitivity to cold pressor pain was increased in opioid addicts compared to healthy controls but remained unchanged during the four-week detoxification program. In contrast, chronic pain patients on a daily morphine dose more than 200 mg developed an increased sensitivity to cold pressor pain at the end of a detoxification program lasting one to two weeks. A study in a very small number of volunteers acutely rendered opioid dependent also documented an increased sensitivity to cold pressor pain during precipitated withdrawal (24). These results echo findings reported in former opioid addicts on methadone. However, whether an increased sensitivity to cold pressor pain can regularly been observed during opioid detoxification remains controversial.

## Patients Undergoing Surgery

A series of studies in patients undergoing surgery suggests that exposure to a high rather than low intraoperative opioid dose is associated with increased pain and/or opioid consumption in the postoperative period (25–29) (Table 2). These findings can be explained by the development of acute OIH in patients exposed to the larger opioid dose. Alternatively, the results could be explained by the development of acute tolerance. The question whether these patients developed acute OIH and/or tolerance cannot be resolved because patients' pain sensitivity before and after the surgery was not formally assessed. However, one study demonstrated that the allodynic and hyperalgesic skin area surrounding the surgical wound was significantly larger in patients exposed to a high rather than low intraoperative opioid dose (28). This result provides direct evidence for aggravated wound hyperalgesia as a consequence of a high opioid dose during surgery. Unfortunately, it is unclear whether aggravated wound hyperalgesia can account for increased resting pain and opioid consumption in the postoperative period.

Not all studies in patients undergoing surgery arrived at the conclusion that the use of a high intraoperative opioid dose is associated with increased postoperative pain and/or opioid consumption (31,32). Differences in total opioid

**Table 2** Studies in Patients Undergoing Surgery

| Reference | Surgery | Intraoperative | | Postoperative | | Remarks |
|---|---|---|---|---|---|---|
| | | Opioid | Dose | Opioid use | Pain | |
| Cooper (26) | Cesarean section | Fentanyl IT | 0 vs. 25 µg | ~60%↑ | ND | $N = 60$; 23-hr observation |
| Chia (30) | Hysterectomy | Fentanyl IV | 1 vs. 22 µg/kg | ~120%↑ | ~30%↑ | $N = 60$; 16-hr observation |
| Guignard (27) | Colectomy | Remifentanil IV | 0.1 vs. 0.3 µg/kg/min for 260 min | ~85%↑ | ~50%↑ | $N = 50$; 24-hr observation |
| Cortinez (31) | Gynecologic | Remifentanil IV | 0.1 vs. 0.23 µg/kg/min for 100 min | ND | ND | $N = 60$; 24-hr observation |
| Joly (28) | Colectomy | Remifentanil IV | 0.05 vs. 0.4 µg/kg/min for 260 min | ~30%↑ | ND[a,b] | $N = 50$; 48-hr observation |
| Lee (32) | Colorectal | Remifentanil IV | N2O vs. 0.17 µg/kg/min for 140 min | ND | ND | $N = 60$; 24-hr observation |
| Crawford (29) | Scoliosis | Remifentanil IV plus MS vs. MS alone | 0.28 µg/kg/min for 460 min[c] | ~30%↑ | ND | $N = 30$; 24-hr observation |

[a]Measures of secondary hyperalgesia were increased (~25%↓ in mechanical pain threshold and 120%↑ in area).
[b]Prevented by intraoperative (0.5 mg/kg → 5 µg/kg/min) and postoperative (2 µg/kg/min for 48 hr) ketamine.
[c]Intraoperative MS consumption was 198 versus 237 µg/kg/min for group R and MS, respectively.
*Abbreviations*: IT, intrathecal; IV, intravenous; ND, not different; N, number of patients.

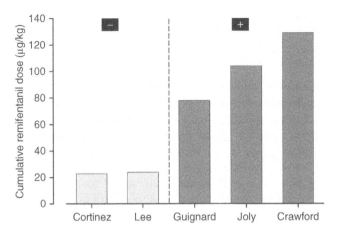

**Figure 1** Some studies in patients undergoing surgery reported increased postoperative pain, and opioid consumption in patients exposed to high rather than low intraoperative opioid doses; findings were compatible with the development of acute opioid-induced hyperalgesia. However, other studies reported negative findings. Authors of the different studies are listed on the *x*-axis. Differences in total opioid exposure during surgery likely explain the discrepant results. Studies using remifentanil and reporting negative results (light gray bars) administered cumulative doses between 20 and 30 µg/kg, whereas studies reporting positive results (dark gray bars) administered cumulative doses between 80 and 120 µg/kg. These findings suggest that OIH develops in dose-dependent fashion and only becomes evident when total opioid exposure is quite high.

exposure during surgery may, however, explain the discrepant results (Fig. 1). For example, studies using remifentanil and reporting negative results administered cumulative doses between 20 and 30 µg/kg, whereas studies reporting positive results administered cumulative doses between 80 and 120 µg/kg. These findings are compatible with the view that acute OIH and/or tolerance develops in a dose-dependent fashion and only becomes evident when total opioid exposure is quite high.

## Experimental Pain Studies in Human Volunteers

Several investigators examined the development of OIH after administering a short-term opioid infusion to human volunteers (33–35). Studies consistently reported that a 30- to 90-minute infusion of remifentanil dose-dependently aggravated preexisting skin hyperalgesia. Aggravated hyperalgesia was observed up to four hours after stopping the infusion. Two studies also assessed sensitivity to heat pain (33,34). Heat-pain sensitivity was not altered after short-term administration of remifentanil. Results of these volunteer studies are consistent with studies in chronic pain and surgical patients and suggest that opioid therapy can aggravate hyperalgesia in skin and surgical wounds but hardly increase pain evoked by brief noxious stimulation of the skin (17,20,28).

## Summary of Clinical Evidence

Studies reporting aggravation of hyperalgesia by opioids, either in human volunteers or in patients undergoing surgery, provide the only direct evidence for the development of OIH in humans (28,33–35).

Considerable indirect evidence for the development of OIH comes from studies documenting either increased sensitivity to cold pressor pain in patients on chronic opioid therapy, or aggravated postoperative pain and increased opioid consumption in patients exposed to high intraoperative opioid doses. However, these studies are limited in several ways. An increased sensitivity to cold pressor pain could be a characteristic of patients vulnerable to develop addictive diseases or requiring opioids for the treatment of chronic pain, rather than being a consequence of opioid therapy. It is also unclear whether an increased sensitivity to cold pressor pain reflects an altered affective response to pain rather than an increased pain sensation. As such, the validity of "cold pressor pain sensitivity" as a marker of OIH will need confirmation from prospective clinical trials. Similarly, increased postoperative pain and opioid consumption in patients exposed to high intraoperative opioid doses could reflect the onset of acute tolerance rather than OIH. Formal assessment of patients' pain sensitivity before and after surgery will be needed to differentiate between acute tolerance and OIH.

Finally, two recent studies using novel pain test paradigms are noteworthy (18,22). These studies documented increased pain on injection of local anesthetics and the less effective suppression of pain by DNIC mechanisms in patients on chronic opioid therapy. While results of these studies will need replication, provided data significantly broaden the body of evidence for the occurrence of OIH in humans.

## OIH with Ultrahigh and Escalating Doses

A series of case reports has described the development of severe allodynia in patients receiving very high and escalating opioid doses, a dosing pattern most commonly observed in the treatment of cancer pain. These reports are discussed in detail in recent reviews (1,2). Patients suffered from widespread tenderness of the skin and soft tissue and experienced episodes of severe pain when touched or gently moved. Allodynic complaints were often accompanied by myoclonic activity. This phenomenon is typically referred to as OIH but may better be labeled opioid-induced allodynia (OIA). Allodynia is characterized by pain to sensory input that normally does not evoke pain (e.g., touch), whereas hyperalgesia is characterized by increased pain to sensory input that normally evokes pain (e.g., heat).

Unlike OIH observed during opioid maintenance therapy, OIA is not mediated by the μ-opioid receptor system. Its expression most likely reflects net excitatory sensory activity resulting from opioid-mediated suppression of gly-cinergic inhibitory neuronal pathways. Escalating the opioid dose worsens the symptoms and administration of an opioid receptor antagonist has no effect. Dose reduction/elimination or opioid rotation offers the most promising thera-peutic approaches to OIA. Opioids with phenantrene structure, such as morphine, have typically been implicated in evoking OIA. This observation provides some rationale for switching to piperidine derivatives such as fentanyl or sufentanil when rotating opioids.

## OIH with Ultralow Doses

The notion that the ultralow doses of opioids can cause hyperalgesia is solely based on studies in animals. These animal studies suggest that excitatory phe-nomena caused by low opioid concentrations gradually give way to analgesic effects as the concentrations rise. Only a single anecdotal report hints toward this type of OIH in humans (1). However, several investigators used a different angle to exploit the idea that ultralow opioid doses could exert hyperalgesic effects. They proposed that blocking these effects with an ultralow dose of an opioid antagonist may enhance net analgesic effects exerted by therapeutic opioid doses.

Results of studies examining whether combining an ultralow dose of an opioid antagonist with an opioid agonist would provide superior analgesia are mixed (36–41). Results are summarized in Table 3.

The majority of studies were conducted in patients undergoing surgery and some reported that addition of ultralow doses of an opioid antagonist enhanced the net analgesic effects, decreased the opioid requirements, and/or reduced the incidence of opioid-mediated side effects. However, other studies found no differences or even decreased analgesic efficacy when adding ultralow doses of an opioid antagonist. Important differences between these studies include the dose and type of administered opioid antagonist, as well as the dosing pattern. Future large-scale clinical studies will need to determine whether coadminis-tration of ultralow doses of an opioid antagonist enhances opioid-mediated analgesia and/or reduces the incidence and severity of opioid side effects. These studies will need to explore a range of antagonist doses to provide a definite answer as to whether an effective dose of ultralow antagonist can be identified in humans.

Recently, the effectiveness of oxycodone combined with an ultralow dose of the opioid antagonist naltrexone (Oxytrex®) has been tested in two separate studies conducted in patients suffering from either osteoarthritis or low back pain (42,43). While superior analgesic effects and a reduced incidence for opioid side effects were reported for Oxytrex, results have to be interpreted cautiously. Oxycodone was dosed four times a day when given alone, whereas Oxytrex was given twice a day. Differences in dosing pattern rather than addition of an ultralow dose of naltrexone could explain observed differences.

**Table 3** Studies Combining Opioids with Ultralow Opioid-Antagonist Doses

| Reference | Patient | Opioid antagonist[a] | Pain | Opioid dose | Opioid side effects[b] | | | | | Remarks |
|---|---|---|---|---|---|---|---|---|---|---|
| | | | | | N | V | P | S | RD | |
| Gan (36) | Hysterectomy | 0.25 µg/kg/hr NX-I | ND | 29%↓ | 44%↓ | 64%↓ | 55%↓ | ND | ND | N = 60; 24-hr-observation |
| | | 1.0 µg/kg/hr NX-I | ND | ND | 57%↓ | 64%↓ | 64%↓ | ND | ND | observation |
| Joshi (37) | Abdominal surgery | 15 µg NM-B | 36%↓ | ND | 42%↓ | ND | 91%↓ | – | – | N = 120; 24-hr-observation |
| | | 25 µg NM-B | 58%↓ | ND | 48%↓ | ND | 91%↓ | – | – | observation |
| Cepeda (38) | Abdominal surgery (∼80%) | 6 µg per 1 mg MS PCA-B | ↑ | ↑ | ND | ND | ND | ND | – | N = 166; 24-hr-observation |
| Cepeda (39) | Abdominal surgery (∼80%) | 0.6 µg per 1 mg MS PCA-B | ND | ND | ND | 21%↓ | 50%↓ | ND | – | N = 265; 24-hr-observation |
| Bijur (40) | Acute pain in ED | 0.1 ng/kg NX-B | ND | ND | ND | ND | – | – | – | N = 156; 4-hr-observation |
| | | 0.01 ng/kg NX-B | ND | ND | ND | ND | – | – | – | observation |
| | | 0.001 ng/kg NX-B | ND | ND | ND | ND | – | – | – | |
| Yeh (41) | Gynecologic surgery | 0.1 µg per 1 mg MS PCA-B | ND | ND | ND | ND | ND | – | – | N = 112; 24-hr-observation |
| | | 1.0 µg per 1 mg MS PCA-B | ND | ND | 59%↓ | ND | ND | – | – | |

[a]NX-I, naloxone infusion; NM-B, nalmefene intravenous bolus; MS PCA-B, morphine bolus with patient-controlled analgesia; NX-B naloxone intravenous bolus.
[b]N, nausea; V, vomiting; P, pruritus; S, sedation; RD, respiratory depression.
*Abbreviations*: ND, no statistically significant difference; N, number of patients.

## CLINICAL PRESENTATION

Three types of OIH have been described in this chapter. OIH observed during opioid maintenance therapy and withdrawal is likely the most relevant type of OIH to clinical medicine. Possible clinical presentations will be discussed in this section. The other two types of OIH are: (*i*) OIH observed in the context of administering very high and escalating opioid doses, which represents a serious problem in affected patients but occurs quite sporadically, and (*ii*) OIH associated with ultralow opioid doses, which may generally render opioid therapy less effective but currently is of unknown clinical significance. The clinical presentation and management of these two types of OIH have briefly been discussed in previous paragraphs.

### Increased Dose Requirements

Opioid therapy can result in a need to increase the dose over time to maintain a desired analgesic effect. Progression of the underlying disease or psychiatric comorbidities are nonpharmacological reasons that can impose as a loss of treatment effect. In the absence of such reasons, the loss of treatment effect is typically attributed to the development of tolerance. However, OIH can also become manifest as a loss of treatment effect. Figure 2 illustrates why both, tolerance and OIH can have the same net effect. Tolerance results from a

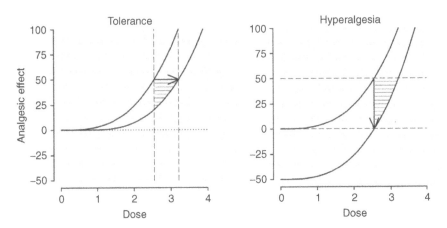

**Figure 2** Tolerance and opioid-induced hyperalgesia (OIH) are pharmacologically distinct phenomena that share the same net effect on dose requirements (stripped area). If tolerance is expressed, decreased drug potency is reflected by a right shift of the dose versus effect relationship as shown in the graph on the left. If OIH is expressed increased pain sensitivity is reflected by a downward shift of the dose versus effect relationship as indicated in the graph on the right. Both tolerance and OIH become clinically apparent as increased dose requirements. Indicated by the stripped area is the apparent net increase in dose that is needed to achieve half maximum analgesic effects.

desensitization of pain signaling pathways to opioids and is pharmacologically characterized by a loss of potency or a right-shift of the dose versus effect relationship. OIH results from sensitization of pain signaling pathways and is characterized by increased pain sensitivity or a downward shift of the dose versus effect relationship. Both, a right-shift and a downward shift of the dose versus effect relationship appear clinically as a loss of treatment effect. The importance of distinguishing between tolerance and OIH becomes evident when considering strategies to overcome the loss in treatment effect. Tolerance may quite simply be addressed by increasing the dose. However, the same intervention may result in aggravated pain in the case of OIH, since opioids are the causative agents.

## Aggravated Pain with Dose Escalation

Several reports described aggravation of cancer pain or postsurgical pain in patients receiving increasing doses of an opioid (44–46). Aggravated clinical pain was not accompanied by overt signs of allodynia and decreased upon opioid dose reduction or substitution with nonopioid analgesics. Paradoxical aggravation of pain after opioid administration and/or dose escalation is the most obvious clinical presentation of OIH.

## Exaggerated Pain Response

Anecdotally, patients on chronic opioid therapy appear to be uniquely sensitive to minor interventions such as an injection, and quickly complain of discomfort. Atypical and heightened pain sensitivity may reflect OIH. For example, patients on chronic opioid therapy and undergoing surgery experience aggravated pain despite consuming larger amounts of pain medications in the postoperative period (47–49). Many of these patients appear to be either in pain or heavily sedated; the therapeutic index of opioids can be markedly reduced in some of these patients. OIH may manifest as a decreased therapeutic window and put patients at increased risk for experiencing serious opioid side effects and/or ineffective pain control.

## The Diagnosis of OIH

Increased opioid requirements or aggravated pain may be manifestations of OIH. However, the development of tolerance, the progression of an underlying disease, or psychiatric comorbidities may similarly impose as a loss of treatment effect. The diagnosis of OIH requires the exclusion of nonpharmacological reasons for increased opioid dose requirements. The question then arises how to best distinguish between OIH and tolerance. In a clinical setting such a distinction may be quite challenging. While not widely used today, quantitative sensory tests specifically assessing a patient's pain sensitivity before and after initiation of opioid therapy may be best suited to separate OIH from tolerance.

In the absence of quantitative sensory data, a patient's history may provide clues. Possible hints include (*i*) pain complaints in excess of those made before initiating opioid therapy, (*ii*) heightened pain sensitivity to minor procedures such as undergoing dental hygiene or intravenous cannulation, and (*iii*) lack of sustained periods of pain relief while on chronic opioid therapy. Finally, a trial of dose escalation can help distinguishing OIH from tolerance. If dose escalation fails relieving pain or even worsens pain, OIH is a likely diagnosis. Dose reduction or complete opioid tapering under careful supervision is a reasonable next step. The partial or complete resolution of pain after taper provides retrospective evidence for OIH.

## STATUS OF THE FIELD

Animal studies provide robust evidence that opioid therapy can be associated with the development of OIH. This matches clinical observations suggesting that patients on chronic opioid therapy can suffer from heightened pain sensitivity or aggravated clinical pain. However, scientific evidence for the development of OIH in humans is limited. At this point, we know with reasonable certainty that opioid therapy can result in exaggerated hyperalgesia. For example, patients undergoing surgery and receiving high intraoperative opioid doses developed aggravated wound hyperalgesia (28). Aggravated hyperalgesia is a concern because this condition may make patients more vulnerable to developing chronic pain conditions (50). However, it is unclear whether aggravated hyperalgesia is associated with increased clinical pain. Interventions attenuating hyperalgesia in other settings do not necessarily decrease spontaneous pain (50). Given the current evidence, OIH could reasonably be portrayed as a condition that renders patients more sensitive to minor traumatic or interventional events. As such, heightened pain sensitivity is a possible side effect associated with opioid therapy. Serious consideration needs to be given to the possibility that OIH may constitute a risk factor for the development of chronic pain.

Most of the scientific evidence generated in humans is indirect in nature. This concern limits the power of some of our most important studies suggesting that OIH may underlay increased clinical pain such as postsurgical pain. Other reasons than OIH can explain observed results. Increased pain in patients undergoing surgery and receiving high intraoperative opioid doses can reflect tolerance rather than OIH. Similarly, increased pain evoked by the cold pressor test in former addicts on methadone or in patients on chronic opioid therapy may reflect a predisposition of subjects with heightened pain sensitivity to use or abuse opioids rather than the onset of OIH. Results obtained with the cold pressor test are further challenged by the fact that investigators using other pain modalities for measuring pain sensitivity could not find evidence for the occurrence of OIH. At this point, it remains unclear whether OIH in humans can account for aggravated clinical pain. While supported by some observational studies, other investigators demonstrated a disconnection between clinical pain and the sensitivity to cold pressor pain. While patients become more sensitive to cold pressor pain, their clinical pain remained unchanged or improved slightly (17,23).

It is reasonable to conclude that OIH can, under some circumstances, be associated with opioid therapy in humans. However, the clinical manifestations and implications of OIH will need further clarification. Well-controlled prospective studies in patients initiated on opioid therapy will need to clarify (*i*) the relationship among opioid dose, therapy duration, and OIH, (*ii*) whether OIH can aggravate clinical pain, (*iii*) whether OIH differentially affects various types of clinical pain (e.g., inflammatory versus neuropathic), (*iv*) whether certain patient populations are at a particular risk for developing OIH, and (*v*) whether OIH is a risk factor for developing chronic pain. A second important endeavor is to gain a better understanding on how results from quantitative sensory tests relate to possible clinical manifestations of OIH. The utility of the cold pressor test as a marker of OIH has been challenged (18). Models evoking heat, electrical, or mechanical pain have failed to detect OIH. Promising alternatives that need validation in the near future are the assessment of DNIC mechanisms and chemically evoked pain (18,22).

While much work needs to done, it is probably safe to suggest that the risk for developing OIH becomes greater as the opioid dose increases (22,23,35). This view favors the conservative use of opioids and certainly discourages from using high or "heroic" opioid doses. Similarly, the use of multimodal analgesic regimens minimizing the reliance on opioids alone is an advisable strategy.

## REFERENCES

1. Angst MS, Clark JD. Opioid-induced hyperalgesia: a qualitative systematic review. Anesthesiology 2006; 104(3):570–587.
2. Chu LF, Angst MS, Clark D. Opioid-induced hyperalgesia in humans: molecular mechanisms and clinical considerations. Clin J Pain 2008; 24(6):479–496.
3. Chang G, Chen L, Mao J. Opioid tolerance and hyperalgesia. Med Clin North Am 2007; 91(2):199–211.
4. Simonnet G, Rivat C. Opioid-induced hyperalgesia: abnormal or normal pain? Neuroreport 2003; 14(1):1–7.
5. Ossipov MH, Lai J, King T, et al. Underlying mechanisms of pronociceptive consequences of prolonged morphine exposure. Biopolymers 2005; 80(2–3):319–324.
6. Fist MB, Frances A, Pincus HA. DSM-IV-TR Guidbook: The Essential Companion to the Diagnostic and Statistical Manual of Mental Disorders. 4th ed. Washington: American Psychiatric Publishing, Inc., 2004:153–155.
7. Himmelsbach CK. The morphine abstinence syndrome, its nature and treatment. Ann Intern Med 1941; 15:829–839.
8. Compton MA. Cold-pressor pain tolerance in opiate and cocaine abusers: correlates of drug type and use status. J Pain Symptom Manage 1994; 9(7):462–473.

9. Compton P, Charuvastra VC, Kintaudi K, et al. Pain responses in methadone-maintained opioid abusers. J Pain Symptom Manage 2000; 20(4):237–245.

10. Compton P, Charuvastra VC, Ling W. Pain intolerance in opioid-maintained former opiate addicts: effect of long-acting maintenance agent. Drug Alcohol Depend 2001; 63(2):139–146.

11. Doverty M, Somogyi AA, White JM, et al. Methadone maintenance patients are cross-tolerant to the antinociceptive effects of morphine. Pain 2001; 93(2):155–163.

12. Doverty M, White JM, Somogyi AA, et al. Hyperalgesic responses in methadone maintenance patients. Pain 2001; 90(1–2):91–96.

13. Dyer KR, Foster DJ, White JM, et al. Steady-state pharmacokinetics and pharma-codynamics in methadone maintenance patients: comparison of those who do and do not experience withdrawal and concentration-effect relationships. Clin Pharmacol Ther 1999; 65(6):685–694.

14. Schall U, Katta T, Pries E, et al. Pain perception of intravenous heroin users on maintenance therapy with levomethadone. Pharmacopsychiatry 1996; 29(5):176–179.

15. Rainville P, Feine JS, Bushnell MC, et al. A psychophysical comparison of sensory and affective responses to four modalities of experimental pain. Somatosens Mot Res 1992; 9:265–277.

16. Pud D, Cohen D, Lawental E, et al. Opioids and abnormal pain perception: new evidence from a study of chronic opioid addicts and healthy subjects. Drug Alcohol Depend 2006; 82(3):218–223.

17. Chu LF, Clark DJ, Angst MS. Opioid tolerance and hyperalgesia in chronic pain patients after one month of oral morphine therapy: a preliminary prospective study. J Pain 2006; 7(1):43–48.

18. Ram KC, Eisenberg E, Haddad M, et al. Oral opioid use alters DNIC but not cold pain perception in patients with chronic pain—new perspective of opioid-induced hyperalgesia. Pain 2008; 139(2):431–438.

19. Hay JL, White JM, Bochner F, et al. Hyperalgesia in opioid-managed chronic pain and opioid-dependent patients. J Pain 2009; 10:316–322.

20. Reznikov I, Pud D, Eisenberg E. Oral opioid administration and hyperalgesia in patients with cancer or chronic nonmalignant pain. Br J Clin Pharmacol 2005; 60(3): 311–318.

21. Fillingim RB, Doleys DM, Edwards RR, et al. Clinical characteristics of chronic back pain as a function of gender and oral opioid use. Spine 2003; 28(2):143–150.

22. Cohen SP, Christo PJ, Wang S, et al. The effect of opioid dose and treatment duration on the perception of a painful standardized clinical stimulus. Reg Anesth Pain Med 2008; 33(3):199–206.

23. Younger J, Barelka P, Carroll I, et al. Reduced cold pain tolerance in chronic pain patients following opioid detoxification. Pain Med 2008; 9(8):1158–1163.

24. Compton P, Athanasos P, Elashoff D. Withdrawal hyperalgesia after acute opioid physical dependence in nonaddicted humans: a preliminary study. J Pain 2003; 4(9): 511–519.

25. Chia YY, Chow LH, Hung CC, et al. Gender and pain upon movement are associated with the requirements for postoperative patient-controlled iv analgesia: a prospective survey of 2,298 Chinese patients. Can J Anaesth 2002; 49(3):249–255.

26. Cooper DW, Lindsay SL, Ryall DM, et al. Does intrathecal fentanyl produce acute cross-tolerance to i.v. morphine? Br J Anaesth 1997; 78(3):311–313.

27. Guignard B, Bossard AE, Coste C, et al. Acute opioid tolerance: intraoperative remifentanil increases postoperative pain and morphine requirement. Anesthesiology 2000; 93:409–417.
28. Joly V, Richebe P, Guignard B, et al. Remifentanil-induced postoperative hyperalgesia and its prevention with small-dose ketamine. Anesthesiology 2005; 103(1): 147–155.
29. Crawford MW, Hickey C, Zaarour C, et al. Development of acute opioid tolerance during infusion of remifentanil for pediatric scoliosis surgery. Anesth Analg 2006; 102(6):1662–1667.
30. Chia YY, Liu K, Wang JJ, et al. Intraoperative high dose fentanyl induces postoperative fentanyl tolerance. Can J Anaesth 1999; 46:872–877.
31. Cortinez LI, Brandes V, Munoz HR, et al. No clinical evidence of acute opioid tolerance after remifentanil-based anaesthesia. Br J Anaesth 2001; 87(6):866–869.
32. Lee LH, Irwin MG, Lui SK. Intraoperative remifentanil infusion does not increase postoperative opioid consumption compared with 70% nitrous oxide. Anesthesiology 2005; 102(2):398–402.
33. Angst MS, Koppert W, Pahl I, et al. Short-term infusion of the mu-opioid agonist remifentanil in humans causes hyperalgesia during withdrawal. Pain 2003; 106:49–57.
34. Hood DD, Curry R, Eisenach JC. Intravenous remifentanil produces withdrawal hyperalgesia in volunteers with capsaicin-induced hyperalgesia. Anesth Analg 2003; 97(3):810–815.
35. Koppert W, Sittl R, Scheuber K, et al. Differential modulation of remifentanil-induced analgesia and postinfusion hyperalgesia by S-ketamine and clonidine in humans. Anesthesiology 2003; 99(1):152–159.
36. Gan TJ, Ginsberg B, Glass PS, et al. Opioid-sparing effects of a low-dose infusion of naloxone in patient-administered morphine sulfate. Anesthesiology 1997; 87(5): 1075–1081.
37. Joshi GP, Duffy L, Chehade J, et al. Effects of prophylactic nalmefene on the incidence of morphine-related side effects in patients receiving intravenous patient-controlled analgesia. Anesthesiology 1999; 90(4):1007–1011.
38. Cepeda MS, Africano JM, Manrique AM, et al. The combination of low dose of naloxone and morphine in PCA does not decrease opioid requirements in the postoperative period. Pain 2002; 96(1–2):73–79.
39. Cepeda MS, Alvarez H, Morales O, et al. Addition of ultralow dose naloxone to postoperative morphine PCA: unchanged analgesia and opioid requirement but decreased incidence of opioid side effects. Pain 2004; 107(1–2):41–46.
40. Bijur PE, Schechter C, Esses D, et al. Intravenous bolus of ultra-low-dose naloxone added to morphine does not enhance analgesia in emergency department patients. J Pain 2006; 7(2):75–81.
41. Yeh YC, Lin TF, Wang CH, et al. Effect of combining ultralow-dose naloxone with morphine in intravenous patient-controlled analgesia: the cut-off ratio of naloxone to morphine for antiemesis after gynecologic surgery. J Formos Med Assoc 2008; 107(6): 478–484.
42. Webster LR, Butera PG, Moran LV, et al. Oxytrex minimizes physical dependence while providing effective analgesia: a randomized controlled trial in low back pain. J Pain 2006; 7(12):937–946.

43. La Vincente SF, White JM, Somogyi AA, et al. Enhanced buprenorphine analgesia with the addition of ultra-low-dose naloxone in healthy subjects. Clin Pharmacol Ther 2008; 83(1):144–152.
44. Vorobeychik Y, Chen L, Bush MC, et al. Improved opioid analgesic effect following opioid dose reduction. Pain Med 2008; 9:724–727.
45. Wilson GR, Reisfield GM. Morphine hyperalgesia: a case report. Am J Hosp Palliat Care 2003; 20:459–461.
46. Guntz E, Talla G, Roman A, et al. Opioid-induced hyperalgesia. Eur J Anaesthesiol 2007; 24:205–207.
47. Carroll IR, Angst MS, Clark JD. Management of perioperative pain in patients chronically consuming opioids. Reg Anesth Pain Med 2004; 29(6):576–591.
48. de Leon-Casasola OA, Lema MJ. Epidural bupivacaine/sufentanil therapy for postoperative pain control in patients tolerant to opioid and unresponsive to epidural bupivacaine/morphine. Anesthesiology 1994; 80(2):303–309.
49. Rapp SE, Ready LB, Nessly ML. Acute pain management in patients with prior opioid consumption: a case-controlled retrospective review. Pain 1995; 61(2):195–201.
50. De Kock M, Lavand'homme P, Waterloos H. 'Balanced analgesia' in the perioperative period: is there a place for ketamine? Pain 2001; 92(3):373–380.

# 4

# Clinical Assessment Tools: Quantitative Sensory Testing

**Robert R. Edwards**

*Department of Anesthesiology, Brigham and Women's Hospital, and Harvard School of Medicine, Boston, Massachusetts, U.S.A.*

## INTRODUCTION

As documented in recent reviews, there is considerable evidence of abnormal pain perception across a broad range of clinical conditions (1). The apparent patterns are generally syndrome-specific, with globally enhanced sensitivity in some conditions (e.g., fibromyalgia), locally diminished sensitivity to pain in other conditions (e.g., diabetic neuropathy), and in some cases a variable mixture of both [e.g., postherpetic neuralgia (PHN)]. This growing body of evidence for alterations in pain perception in many clinical populations has stimulated a great deal of interest in experimental pain assessment, or quantitative sensory testing (QST), and its potential application in the clinical setting. However, it is also important to note that individual variability in pain perception is substantial even within nonclinical samples (2,3), and QST can be used to study these individual differences in pain sensitivity and pain processing. This chapter provides an overview of the methodology and clinical relevance of QST, highlighting its applications in clinical settings. Throughout the chapter, the terms QST and experimental pain assessment will be used interchangeably to describe a variety of psychophysical procedures that include multiple methods for evaluating responses to standardized noxious stimuli.

## HISTORY

Experimental pain assessment dates back well over a century, when individual differences in pain responses were initially reported in scientific settings (4). In retrospect, most of the early studies used fairly rudimentary testing procedures, with electricity, mechanical pressure, or radiant heat applied in a manner that was rarely standardized with much precision. Moreover, validated pain response scales were rarely employed in those early studies. In the 1950s the advent of sensory decision theory, or signal detection theory (SDT), set the stage for modern-day QST (5). While later critiques of SDT cogently questioned apologists' claims that the SDT methodology could reliably differentiate "pure" sensory processes from responses driven by other factors (6), SDT provided a solid foundation for the multidimensional assessment of experimental pain responses.

In the 1980s, QST methods were integral to early studies assessing pain-related brain activation (7). Such studies generally require fairly precise quantification of nociceptive input, and the success of QST in this arena is evidenced, in part, by the recent deluge of functional MRI studies assessing the central nervous system correlates of normal and abnormal pain perception (8,9). QST has also been instrumental in facilitating the psychophysical study of endogenous pain-modulatory processes. For example, increasing number of studies assess the effects of a heterotopic noxious conditioning stimulus on a phasic noxious stimulus; the resultant inhibition of the phasic noxious stimulus is termed diffuse noxious inhibitory controls (DNIC) (10), and these endogenous inhibitory processes appear to be impaired, or to function suboptimally, in some groups of patients (11). In addition, recent work suggests that QST-assessed individual differences in DNIC are prospectively associated with long-term postoperative pain; those with the least effective DNIC systems reported more severe and long-lasting pain following thoracic surgery (12). Finally, in recent years, attention has been turned to the potential of QST to aid in clinical diagnosis and treatment selection, as we elucidate in sections below (1). In particular, the German Research Network on Neuropathic Pain has been instrumental in standardizing QST methods and applying them to large samples of neuropathic pain patients. This group is beginning to publish normative data from their samples, which will be extraordinarily useful in future studies that attempt to classify and subgroup patients with neuropathic pain (13,14).

## QST METHODS

QST extends the traditional neurological examination of sensory function by using psychophysical procedures and an array of stimulus modalities to assess the functional capacity of primary afferent fibers and indirectly and non-invasively gain information about spinal and supraspinal processing of information related to noxious stimulation. Below, the methods involving the various modalities of experimental pain assessment will be briefly described. For a more thorough description of these methods, interested readers are referred to additional previously published articles in this area (13–16).

## Mechanical Pain

The most typical methods for inducing painful mechanical stimulation are the variable-pressure and constant-pressure algometers. For the variable-pressure algometer, a probe is pressed against an area of skin while applying increasing pressure at a constant rate, usually around 1 kg/sec, until a subjective criterion, such as pain tolerance or threshold, is achieved (15). It is important to standardize, within a given study, the rate of pressure increase, as this variable has an influence on pain thresholds (16). The Forgione–Barber pressure dolorimeter, an example of a constant-pressure algometer, applies constant painful pressure to an area of skin for a specified duration or until a subjective criterion is reached (17). Mechanical stimulation has been primarily used to assess pain thresholds over large muscles and joints, although in principle these pressure algometers may be applied to any region of the body. It should be noted that there are wide variations in mechanical pain sensitivity across body sites, necessitating, in some cases, access to anatomic location-specific normative data (18). Recent technological innovations utilize computer-controlled mechanical stimulators, which allows more precise monitoring and calibration of stimulation, enhancing reliability of the technique and eliminating interexaminer variability in factors such as the rate of pressure increase (19).

Smaller-diameter punctuate stimulators are also widely utilized to study mechanical pain. In particular, von Frey filaments are often used in the assessment of hyperalgesia and allodynia, particularly in the context of neuropathic pain. (13,20). Punctate, or pinprick, stimulation has also been used as a form of fiber-selective mechanical stimulation as it is believed to activate predominantly the Aδ primary afferents and produces a sensation that is generally reported as "first pain" (21). Recent recommendations for QST include use of both blunt and punctuate mechanical probes, which allows a full assessment of both A and C fiber function, as well as both superficial and deep nociceptors (13). The German Research Network on Neuropathic Pain also utilizes such punctate mechanical stimulators to investigate temporal summation, or windup, of pain (described in more detail in a later section), in which repetitive noxious stimuli evoke an increasing percept of pain over time (13,14).

## Thermal Pain

While many of the early studies of thermal pain perception utilized radiant heat, the most common modern methodologies involve laser stimulation or the administration of heat using a contact thermode. In terms of laser stimulation, most studies involve application of short-duration pulses (e.g., 20–200 msec), or trains of pulses, from a $CO_2$ laser, which evoke a pricking pain sensation, with many researchers concurrently measuring evoked potentials using electroencephalography (EEG) (22). The Peltier thermode is perhaps the most widely used modern-day devise for thermal pain stimulation, primarily due to its ease of use and because it allows for precise control of the application of heat and cold pain stimuli with a natural quality of sensation (15). The delivery of contact heat stimuli activates both A$\delta$ fibers, where the evoked sensation corresponds to the first pain, and C-fibers, which mediate a burning "second pain" sensation. In general, slow heating with a contact thermode gives a preferential activation of C-fibers and the best evaluation of second pain (23,24). Additionally, as outlined by the German Research Network on Neuropathic Pain, contact thermodes may also be used to investigate responses to nonpainful thermal stimuli (e.g., warmth thresholds, cool thresholds, etc.), which provides important additional information that is especially relevant to the diagnosis, classification, and characterization of neuropathic pain symptoms (for additional detail, see Refs. 13 and 14, and Fig. 1).

Other QST techniques that have been employed to measure thermal nociception include freeze lesions and burn injuries, both of which involve a temperature-dependent tissue-damaging stimulus that results in hyperalgesia (25). These experimental pain models are frequently employed in testing analgesics (26), and are generally considered good models of the primary and secondary hyperalgesia often observed in the context of acute injury and neuropathic pain. They are less commonly used than many of the other techniques described here, probably because they do involve at least some tissue damage. In contrast, many other QST methods are attractive in part because they are nondamaging and produce only transient pain that rarely outlasts the stimulus itself.

Finally, the cold pressor test (CPT) is a classic thermal assessment technique that involves immersion of an extremity, most often the hand or foot, into a very cold water bath (usually with a temperature between 0°C and 5°C). The pain produced during a CPT builds quickly to a peak and can be maintained for minutes, making this a generally more tonic pain induction technique than other thermal stimuli. The CPT does produce substantial pressor responses in most individuals, and is a potent physiological challenge, as reflected by the fact that most QST studies of neuroendocrine responses to pain use a CPT task to stimulate cortisol responses (27). Recent work from our laboratory has also suggested that the CPT, in addition to provoking increases in circulating levels of cortisol, can produce increases in circulating levels of proinflammatory cytokines, making it a useful stimulation tool for investigating inter-relationships between pain and inflammatory processes (28). Notably, recent evidence also indicates that preoperative cold pressor ratings have been shown to be predictive of postoperative pain ratings, suggesting the clinical relevance of individual differences in CPT responses (29,30).

## Electrical Pain

Electrical pain stimulation is one of the oldest forms of QST, and remains in use till today in many laboratories. Notably, electrical stimulation has been criticized as a pain induction technique on the grounds that (*i*) it concurrently stimulates all

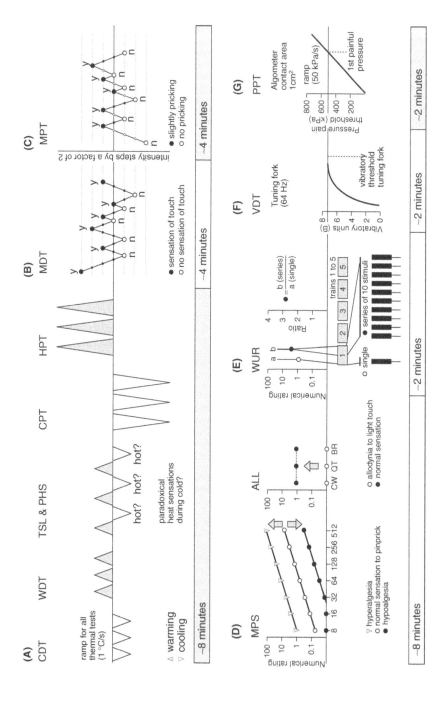

nerve fibers, not just nociceptors, and so is quite nonselective and (*ii*) activation of primary afferents occurs directly by the transfer of electrical energy, effectively bypassing transduction within the nociceptors. However, electrical stimulation does offer extremely precise control over stimulus intensity and timing, which can be an appealing feature in many situations, and it is widely used in the assessment of nociceptive reflexes such as the RIII reflex. In a number of studies, assessing the RIII reflex has allowed investigators to illuminate the associations between spinal processing of nociceptive input and concurrent subjective pain scores (31,32). Indeed, recent RIII studies have documented associations between psychosocial processes and nociceptive processes, one of the common areas of application of QST (33,34). Other electrical QST studies have utilized stimulation of tooth pulp to evaluate psychological interventions (e.g., hypnosis, relaxation training) and their effects on pain responses (35).

## Ischemic Pain

The tourniquet test and the modified submaximal effort tourniquet test have been used for decades in various experimental pain studies to assess ischemic pain (36). In brief, blood flow to an extremity (e.g., the arm) is occluded during isometric muscle exercise, producing local ischemia and consequent ischemic

---

**Figure 1** Battery of QST responses measured by the German Research Network on Neuropathic Pain. The standardized QST protocol assesses 13 parameters in seven test procedures (**A–G**). All procedures are presented including a time frame for testing over one area. (**A**) Thermal testing comprises detection and pain thresholds for cold, warm, or hot stimuli (C- and A-Δ fiber mediated): CDT, WDT, number of PHSs during the TLS procedures for alternating warm and cold stimili, CPT, and HPT. (**B**) MDT test for A-β fiber function using von Frey filaments. (**C**) MPT test for A-Δ-fiber mediated hyper- or hypoalgesia to pinprick stimuli. (**D**) Stimulus-response-functions: MPS for pinprick stimuli, and dynamic mechanical allodynia (ALL) assess A-Δ-mediated sensitivity to sharp stimuli (pinprick), and also A-β fiber–mediated pain sensitivity to stroking light touch (CW, QT, BR, brush). (**E**) WUR compares the numerical ratings within five trains of a single pinprick stimulus (a) with a series (b) of 10 repetitive pincrick stimuli to calculate WUR as the ratio: b/a. (**F**) VDT tests for A-β fiber function using a Rydel–Seiffer 64 Hz tuning fork. (**G**) PPT is the only test for deep pain sensitivity, most probably mediated by muscle C- and A-Δ fibers. For details regarding the testing procedures also see section "QST Methods". *Abbreviations*: CDT, cold detection threshold; WDT, warm detection threshold; PHS, paradoxical heat sensations; TSL, thermal sensory limen procedures; CPT, cold pain threshold; HPT, heat pain threshold; MDT, mechanical detection threshold; MPT, mechanical pain threshold; MPS, mechanical pain sensitivity; CW, cotton wisp; QT, cotton wool tip; BR, brush; WUR, wind-up ratio; VDP, vibration detection threshold; PPT, pressure pain threshold. *Source*: From Ref. 13.

pain. Of all the experimental pain models, this is perhaps most phenomeno-logically similar to musculoskeletal clinical pain (37). The tourniquet test has been used in experimental settings to assess the analgesic efficacy of drugs as well as to induce DNIC (38–40). Moreover, ischemic pain has been shown to be more sensitive than other experimental pain modalities to clinical variables such as menstrual cycle phase (41) and the severity of ongoing chronic pain (42).

## Chemical Pain

Pain stimulation by chemical means involves, in most cases, injection of algo-genic substances such as hypertonic saline into the skin or muscle, or topical application on the skin of histamine or capsaicin. Chemical stimulation is per-haps the least-employed QST technique, but it has been gaining popularity in recent years. There are three major means of painful chemical stimulation, the first of which includes intradermal injection or topical application of capsaicin, which evokes cutaneous pain and subsequent hyperalgesia. This model has been used to test analgesic effects in the context of neuropathic pain. In particular, some studies have quantified the extent of secondary hyperalgesia following standardized topical capsaicin application, and have utilized the resultant data as an index of spinal processing of nociceptive input, as in studies of putative neuropathic pain-relieving medications (43–45). The second chemical QST modality, similar to the capsaicin model, involves the use of mustard oil applied to the skin, which produces inflammation and hyperalgesia and has been used as a model for inflammatory pain (21). Finally, infusion of hypertonic saline into a muscle or joint produces a tonic, aching pain that has been used in recent neuroimaging studies to assess CNS processing of deep tissue pain (46,47).

## Additional QST Techniques: Temporal Summation

A number of QST studies have employed repeated application of noxious stimuli in order to study the temporal summation of pain, a phenomenon linked with central sensitization-like processes (48–50). The assessment of temporal summa-tion involves rapidly applying a series of identical noxious stimuli and determining the increase in pain across trials; animal studies have suggested that temporal summation occurs centrally in second-order wide dynamic range (WDR) spinal neurons in the spinal cord (50). The phenomenon of temporal summation has demonstrated importance in our understanding of pain mechanisms in several arenas. For example, amplified temporal summation of pain has been observed in several common chronic pain conditions in which part of the pathophysiology of the disorder is thought to involve a maladaptive degree of sensitization to pain, such conditions include fibromyalgia (51), temporomandibular joint disorder (TMD) (52) and other myofascial pain conditions (53,54). Moreover, the onset of neuropathic pain is often associated with the observation of abnormally enhanced temporal summation of pain (55,56), and the modulation of temporal summation involves the activity of descending pain-inhibitory systems, which play crucial roles in pain processing (57).

## APPLICATIONS OF QST

### Illuminate Factors Influencing Pain Perception

Multiple biopsychosocial variables can influence the perception of pain. Some of these factors are modifiable, while others generally are not. With respect to the latter category, for example, results of studies using experimental pain assessment indicate that sex and gender-related factors affect the perception and report in multiple ways (58,59). In addition, there are significant age-related differences in pain responses (37), as well as ethnic differences (60). In addition to documenting the influence of demographic variables on pain, QST can also be used to study the impact of psychosocial and behavioral processes. In general, while clinical studies have indicated that cognition, mood, and other psychosocial factors are correlated with chronic pain outcomes (61), it is laboratory studies that have indicated causal associations between such variables and the perception and report of pain. For example, experimental induction of positive moods can reduce pain sensitivity, while negative mood induction enhances pain sensitivity (62–64), suggesting a direct link between mood and pain responses. As a second example, other researchers have used QST to assess the directionality of the associations between pain and sleep, reporting that not only can noxious stimulation disrupt sleep (65), but the disruption of normal sleep can interfere with endogenous pain-inhibitory processes (66). Thus, QST is a tremendous boon to researchers who wish to study the direction and nature of psychosocial and behavioral influences on nociceptive processing.

QST has also been applied to evaluate differences in pain perception and pain processing between clinical populations and healthy controls (67). Such research has important implications regarding the pathophysiology of pain conditions and may ultimately be used to generate a system of mechanism-based diagnosis, which would inform treatment decisions (68). Indeed, a generalized enhancement of sensitivity to painful stimuli, which may suggest involvement of central mechanisms, is well documented in fibromyalgia (69), temporomandibular disorders (53), pelvic pain syndromes (70), abdominal pain (71), and headache disorders (72). Thus, generalized hyperalgesia may serve as a marker for certain pain syndromes, though it is unclear whether this hypersensitivity precedes or is consequent to the onset of chronic pain.

Finally, QST has been instrumental in facilitating the development of a literature on the genetic aspects of pain. A rapidly growing animal literature documents the substantial contribution of genotype to pain sensitivity and pain susceptibility (73). Human studies have now confirmed that certain SNPs (single nucleotide polymorphisms) are associated with differing profiles of opioid receptor binding in the central nervous system (47). Additionally, a recent human research on a number of pain-relevant genes has used QST to demonstrate that genotype impacts both pain sensitivity and clinical pain responses, including the development of a persistent pain condition (74,75). One currently unanswered question concerns the degree of heritability of pain sensitivity, which a recent human study using three QST modalities estimated at between 22% and 46% across three pain modalities (76). These studies all suggest a potentially strong influence of genetic factors in nociceptive processing, and highlight the vital role of employing QST in the translation of animal genetic findings to clinical studies of human patients.

## Improving the Assessment of Clinical Pain

QST can be used to improve the assessment of clinical pain severity, through methods such as matching the intensity of an experimental pain stimulus to clinical pain intensity. In general, in clinical settings, pain severity is assessed using numerical scales, which are often difficult to interpret and may not be comparable across patients. Incorporating QST, patients can be asked to match an experimental pain stimulus to their clinical pain, which provides a more quantifiable index of clinical pain by locating it within an individualized continuum from pain threshold to pain tolerance (77). Findings from this body of research have indicated that patients apply rating scales consistently across experimental and clinical pain modalities, that their actual match points are similar to what would be predicted from psychophysical stimulus-response functions, and that QST is useful in quantifying where on a patient's individual continuum of pain (i.e., from threshold to tolerance), a particular clinical pain experience falls. Overall, QST, in concert with validated scaling methods, provides a valuable index of clinical pain that is anchored to a defined noxious stimulus, and also provides an indication of how consistently individual patients rate pain across stimulus modalities (78).

## Predicting Risk for Future Pain

Among the most clinically applicable uses of QST are findings that responses to standardized noxious stimuli can prospectively predict the course of pain complaints, or the future risk for developing pain. Several recent studies have examined preoperative experimental pain responses as predictors of postoperative pain. Among individuals undergoing limb amputation, preamputation pressure pain thresholds were significantly inversely correlated with postamputation stump pain and phantom pain (79). In addition, preoperative thermal QST responses predicted postoperative pain scores at rest and during activity in women undergoing cesarean section (80). Other investigations have produced comparable results. Following anterior cruciate ligament repair, preoperative ratings of an intense noxious thermal stimulus were strongly correlated with joint pain ratings for several weeks postsurgery (81), though pain thresholds were not generally predictive. Finally, preoperative cold pain tolerance predicted postoperative pain after laparoscopic cholecystectomy, even after controlling for neuroticism (30).

Taken together, these findings identify suprathreshold experimental pain responses as important predictors of acute pain intensity following surgical procedures; additional long-term prospective studies will be necessary to evaluate QST as a predictor of chronic pain following surgery. The observed predictive relationships are often quite strong, for example, in the study of acute pain following cesarean section by Granot et al. (80), preoperative ratings of noxious thermal stimuli prospectively predicted up to 54% of the variance in the severity of postoperative pain. Moreover, several recent studies have noted that presurgical QST responses can predict even long-term pain complaints postsurgery. In a recent report on 63 patients with knee osteoarthritis, who were tested preoperatively and followed up at 18 months after undergoing total knee replacement, lower preoperative electrical pain thresholds independently predicted more severe long-term knee pain (82). A recent study of thoracotomy patients also indicated that those with the least effective DNIC systems, assessed preoperatively, reported more severe and long-lasting pain up to six months after surgery (12). Several longitudinal studies in patients with TMD have also offered support for the important role of psychophysical pain responses as markers for long-term pain outcomes. In patients with TMD, enhanced sensitivity to mechanical stimulation has been specifically associated with the persistence and spread of TMD pain (83,84), and in a recent prospective cohort study of initially healthy young women, higher basal pain sensitivity was associated with a greater than twofold increase in the risk of developing TMD over the three-year course of the study (75,85).

## Subgrouping of Pain Patients

Diagnostic validity is an important issue in the classification of chronic pain, and many have argued that the current symptom-driven taxonomy for classifying pain complaints is inadequate (68). Indeed, QST has already become a valuable tool in diagnosing peripheral nerve disorders (86), especially early small-fiber neuropathies that are not readily detected by standard nerve conduction studies (87). Additional applications include the classification of sensory abnormalities in central pain states associated with conditions such as multiple sclerosis or stroke (88), though it is important to emphasize that QST abnormalities are not specific to neuropathic pain states (87). QST is routinely used and widely accepted in the diagnosis of painful conditions that include tenderness or enhanced pain sensitivity as part of the diagnostic criteria (e.g., fibromyalgia), and an increasing preponderance of research suggests that maladaptively amplified CNS pain processing, as assessed by QST, is likely to play a substantial etiological role in a broad spectrum of regional and widespread pain conditions (89,90).

Recent studies have examined QST findings within many chronic pain disorders. For example, Pappagallo et al. (91) detected increased thresholds to heat and cold pain in the affected area of thoracic but not trigeminal PHNpatients, suggesting the potential for the differentiation of PHN syndromes based on distinct pathophysiological mechanisms. Similar findings in terms of sensory change and alterations in pain detection thresholds were reported with patients diagnosed with interstitial cystitis (92). Kleinbohl et al. (93) found that responses to phasic and tonic heat pain not only distinguished chronic pain patients from healthy controls but also discriminated among types of chronic pain (e.g., headache, back pain) with good sensitivity and specificity. Finally, QST and psychosocial measures were used to distinguish three subgroups of FM patients, in whom, it was hypothesized, different pain-maintaining mechanisms were operative (e.g., central sensitization vs. psychological distress) (94). Correspondingly, QST used in conjunction with other relevant neurophysiological tests has been shown to increase diagnostic accuracy. For instance, compared to clinical testing alone, the combination of nerve conduction recordings and thermal QST increased the diagnostic yield to 100% in patients with long-standing postsurgical trigeminal sensory alteration and neuropathy (95,96). Thus, these QST methods seem to provide enhanced specificity for characterizing sensory dysfunction in patients who experience injury and subsequent pain conditions. Collectively, these studies hint that QST could be useful in creating an improved pain classification system that might be based on pathophysiological mechanisms, and which could have substantial prognostic value.

In general, a number of researchers have expressed the hope that QST will aid in the mechanism-based diagnosis of pain, particularly neuropathic pain. For example, QST can be quite valuable, in patients with a variety of neuropathic conditions, in differentiating between such mechanisms as sensory deafferentation, central sensitization, or peripheral sensitization. The German Research Network on Neuropathic Pain has been instrumental in promulgating a standardized set of QST methods, and they have published some normative data for patients and controls as well (13,14). For examples of the type of QST-based differentiation of pain syndromes and the mechanism-based interpretation of somatosensory dysfunction that the German Network has envisioned (Figs. 2 and 3) (13,14).

## Assessing and Predicting Treatment Outcomes

Several investigators have evaluated experimental pain responses as predictors of outcomes following pain-relieving treatments. In a study of multidisciplinary treatment for chronic pain, women with higher pretreatment pain tolerance (assessed using a test of ischemic pain responses) showed greater improvements in pain and activity level than women with lower pain tolerance (97). Similarly, among vulvar vestibulitis patients, pretreatment ratings of suprathreshold thermal pain predicted both choice of treatment and subsequent treatment outcomes (98). Women who were less sensitive on thermal QST testing were more likely

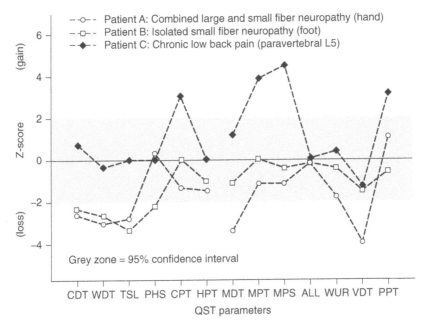

**Figure 2** Example of the variety of sensory findings evident in different pain conditions, using findings from the German Research Network on Neuropathic Pain. Z-score QST profiles of patients undergoing the battery of tests employed by the German Research Network on Neuropathic Pain. Patient A has a combined small and large-fiber neuropathy in the hand. The profile reveals a broad loss of sensory function. Patient B has symptoms of bilateral burning pain in her feet and ankles, and has a small-fiber sensory neuropathy with preservation of large-fiber function. Patient C has chronic low back pain and shows enhanced sensitivity (e.g., a gain of function) to noxious stimuli. *Source*: From Ref. 13.

to choose surgery as a treatment and, across treatments, showed greater reductions in pelvic pain than women with higher heat pain ratings. Finally, animal and human studies have specifically assessed the associations between pain sensitivity and opioid analgesia. For example, a growing animal literature suggests that mice with lower basal heat pain thresholds (i.e., more heat pain-sensitive mice) evidence less analgesia in response to exogenous administration of opioids (99,100). Multiple human studies have at least partially replicated these animal findings, reporting that a higher tolerance for electrical pain at baseline was associated with greater morphine analgesia in an experimental pain model among healthy adults (74), and that a higher presurgical tolerance for pressure pain was correlated with less postoperative morphine consumption following lower abdominal surgery (101). Finally, our group reported that in patients with PHN, higher pretreatment heat pain thresholds were associated with more pain reduction and relief during opioid treatment (102).

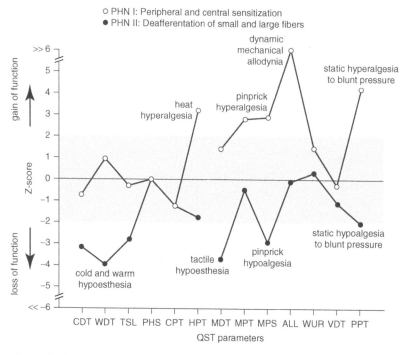

○ PHN I: Peripheral and central sensitization
● PHN II: Deafferentation of small and large fibers

**Figure 3** Example of individual differences in pain mechanisms in patients with the same disorder, from the German Research Network on Neuropathic Pain. Z-score sensory profiles of two patients suffering from PHN. The patient labeled PHN I shows a predominant gain of sensory function consistent with a combination of peripheral and central sensitization. The patient labeled PHN II shows a predominant loss of sensory function consistent with a combined small and large-fiber sensory deafferentation. *Abbreviation*: PHN, postherpetic neuralgia. *Source*: From Ref. 14.

QST can also be used as an outcome measure to document treatment-related changes in somatosensory function. Recently, Kosek and Ordeberg reported thermal hyperalgesia, mechanical hyperalgesia, and deficient pain inhibition in osteoarthritis patients at baseline, but showed that these conditions normalize following successful pain-relieving surgery (39,103). Other researchers have also addressed this issue by studying QST responses separately in treatment responders and nonresponders. In an analgesic trial in fibroymalgia, patients who showed a 50% or greater reduction in clinical pain intensity also showed increases in pressure pain threshold and tolerance, while nonresponders showed no changes in mechanical pain sensitivity (104). Similarly, in a study of amitriptyline treatment for irritable bowel syndrome, gastrointestinal (GI) pain was reduced and visceral pain sensitivity (i.e., the pain threshold to rectal distention) was increased (105); in this study, changes in pain sensitivity closely paralleled changes in clinical pain ($r = -0.71$). Collectively, treatment-related normalization of pain perception is observed only when clinical pain is reduced, suggesting that the QST measure may be a sensitive index of treatment outcome.

## Assessing Opioid-Induced Hyperalgesia

QST has a clear role in the documentation and evaluation of opioid-induced hyperalgesia. Unlike clinical pain, which is subject to daily variability in response to dozens of factors, the use of standardized noxious stimuli permits quantification of changes in pain sensitivity as a function of pharmacologic treatment. A number of studies have used QST to examine long-term opioid-related changes in the perception of pain. For example, individuals with a history of opioid abuse who are maintained on methadone show reduced pain tolerance and enhanced sensitivity to a variety of modalities of painful stimuli, suggesting a long-term sensitization or hyperalgesic process as a consequence of chronic opiate use (106–108). In addition, individuals chronically consuming opioids report greater postoperative pain despite aggressive use of acute opioid dosing (109). Finally, multiple human studies (110) have demonstrated that short-acting opioids such as remifentanil produce hyperalgesia in healthy volunteers (111,112) and following perioperative administration in patients undergoing surgery (113,114). These findings of remifentanil-induced hyperalgesia are generally established by using QST methods to establish an individual's basal pain sensitivity, and then evaluating pain responses at repeated intervals following a dose of remifentanil. Paralleling the animal data, an initial analgesic response is generally followed by an eventual hyperalgesic response, though it is noteworthy that individual differences in opioid analgesia and hyperalgesia are substantial. Given that opioid-induced hyperalgesia is considered a crucial potential mechanism underlying the failure of opioids to relieve chronic pain in many individuals, the numbers of applications and uses of QST in this area are likely to increase (110). Indeed, recent work has used QST to investigate reductions in DNIC as a potential mechanism contributing to opioid-induced hyperalgesia in patients with chronic pain (115).

## Studying Pain Processing in the Brain

Over the past several decades, explosive growth in the field of functional neuroimaging of pain has been observed (8,9). A thorough treatment of this literature is well beyond the scope of the present chapter, but some important points bear mentioning here. First, nearly all of these studies utilize experimental pain stimuli (even if the subjects are experiencing clinical pain) in order to precisely quantify the degree of applied stimulation and to study the central nervous system pathways underlying normal and abnormal pain perceptions. Second, QST methodologies can be utilized in conjunction with neuroimaging to assess such complex biopsychosocial aspects of the pain experience as anticipation of pain (116) and placebo analgesia (117). Finally, many new drugs are being tested using fMRI and experimental pain assessment to determine the drug's effects on specific regions within the pain neuromatrix (9,118), highlighting a broad clinical applicability of combining QST and methodologies such as functional MRI.

## ADVANTAGES AND LIMITATIONS OF QST

The principal advantage of QST is the high level of stimulus control that can be exerted by investigators, a situation that obviously does not pertain to clinical pain. For instance, the anatomical site and tissue depth stimulated can be controlled and varied using experimental pain induction procedures. In a recent QST study, Giamberardino et al. (119) examined responses to electrical pain delivered to three anatomical sites (arm, leg, and abdomen) and at three different tissue depths (skin, subcutis, and muscle) across the menstrual cycle in dysmenorrheic compared to pain-free women. Greater group differences emerged with increasing tissue depth, with the largest effect observed for stimulation of the abdominal muscle. Furthermore, a subsequent study by another research group indicating that remifentanil produced greater analgesia for electrical pain applied to muscle than to skin (120), again demonstrating the value of stimulating at different body sites and tissue depths. QST also provides control over many other stimulus characteristics, including temporal parameters and stimulus intensity. Thus, experimentally evoked pain provides much greater flexibility for addressing both mechanistic and clinical questions of interest. Another clear advantage of QST is the ability to study responses in both healthy and clinical populations. QST methodologies allow investigators to compare responses to identical stimuli in healthy individuals and those with clinical pain disorders (121–123), an approach that has shown broad applicability in elucidating the pathophysiology underlying many clinical conditions, which may ultimately lead to more effective diagnosis and treatment.

The primary disadvantage of QST has been its failure to capture the sensory and especially the affective qualities of clinical pain. Indeed, experimentally induced pain is by nature transient and is not associated with tissue damage or with a high degree of threat to the integrity of the organism. Thus, important psychosocial processes such as catastrophizing may relate strongly to clinical pain but only weakly to experimental pain (124). However, some experimental pain stimuli are capable of producing pain responses that may be quite clinically relevant. As discussed above, temporal summation of thermal pain is believed to reflect some of the neural mechanisms important in certain inflammatory and neuropathic pain states (125,126). Also, some experimental pain tasks are capable of producing more tonic, deeper pain, which may more closely resemble many forms of clinical pain. For example, the submaximal effort tourniquet procedure produces long-lasting ischemic arm pain, which elicits robust affective responses (127), and cold pressor stimulation evokes both psychological responses such as catastrophizing, and physiological responses such as increases in serum levels of cortisol and inflammatory markers (28).

Finally, another experimental pain stimulus, infusion of hypertonic saline (128), may also be highly clinically relevant. Indeed, the infusion of hypertonic saline into masseter muscle in healthy controls produced sensory and affective pain responses that were statistically indistinguishable from the clinical pain reported by patients with persistent facial pain (129).

## CONCLUSION AND SUMMARY

Many of the same factors shaping responses to experimental painful stimuli also contribute to the experience of clinical pain, making QST a valuable tool with which to study many biopsychosocial aspects of pain. However, QST has not yet become a standard component of clinical pain evaluation. While there are some practical barriers, including time, cost, and the use of specialized equipment, it is anticipated that QST will become an increasingly common pain assessment tool, advancing the understanding and management of a wide variety of painful disorders (13). For example, future studies may determine whether QST can be used to determine probable needs for analgesic dosing (e.g., in postsurgical pain models), and whether this application of QST improves outcomes (130). In the coming years, QST may be incorporated into an increasing breadth of clinical and research settings, especially in conjunction with other rapidly developing subfields of clinical pain research, such as pain genetics and functional neuroimaging.

The standardized administration of noxious stimuli under controlled conditions is becoming increasingly common within clinical pain research. A number of recent studies have suggested that quantitative sensory testing, or experimental pain assessment, is quite valuable in identifying pain mechanisms and elucidating individual differences in the experience of pain among both healthy adults and patients with painful conditions. Moreover, quantitative sensory testing techniques have proven themselves useful in the assessment of opioid-induced hyperalgesia. Collectively, the findings reviewed within this chapter suggest that experimental pain responses relate to clinical pain report and potentially to pain treatment outcomes across a variety of samples. For example, experimental pain assessment may be useful in quantifying an individual's future risk for developing chronic pain, or in determining how effective treatment with opioids is likely to be for a given person. The clinical application of quantitative sensory testing can be expected to increase in the future, as it is noninvasive, relatively easy to administer, and provides important prognostic and diagnostic information.

## REFERENCES

1. Edwards RR, Sarlani E, Wesselmann U, et al. Quantitative assessment of experimental pain perception: multiple domains of clinical relevance. Pain 2005; 114(3): 315–319.
2. Gracely R. Studies of pain in human subjects. In: Wall P, Melzack R, eds. Textbook of Pain. New York: Churchill Livingstone, 1999:385–407.

3. Fillingim RB. Individual differences in pain responses. Curr Rheumatol Rep 2005; 7(5):342–347.
4. Nakamura Y, Chapman CR. Measuring pain: an introspective look at introspection. Conscious Cogn 2002; 11(4):582–592.
5. Clark WC. Pain sensitivity and the report of pain: an introduction to sensory decision theory. Anesthesiology 1974; 40(3):272–287.
6. Rollman G. Signal detection theory measurement of pain: a review and critique. Pain 1977; 3:187–211.
7. Bromm B, Scharein E. Principal component analysis of pain-related cerebral potentials to mechanical and electrical stimulation in man. Electroencephalogr Clin Neurophysiol 1982; 53:94–103.
8. Borsook D, Becerra LR. Breaking down the barriers: fMRI applications in pain, analgesia and analgesics. Mol Pain 2006; 2:30.
9. Borsook D, Becerra L. Functional imaging of pain and analgesia—a valid diagnostic tool? Pain 2005; 117(3):247–250.
10. Kraus E, Le Bars D, Besson JM. Behavioral confirmation of "diffuse noxious inhibitory controls" (DNIC) and evidence for a role of endogenous opiates. Brain Res 1981; 206:495–499.
11. Lautenbacher S, Rollman GB. Possible deficiencies of pain modulation in fibromyalgia. Clin J Pain 1997; 13(3):189–196.
12. Yarnitsky D, Crispel Y, Eisenberg E, et al. Prediction of chronic postoperative pain: pre-operative DNIC testing identifies patients at risk. Pain 2008; 138(1):22–28.
13. Rolke R, Magerl W, Campbell KA, et al. Quantitative sensory testing: a comprehensive protocol for clinical trials. Eur J Pain 2006; 10(1):77–88.
14. Rolke R, Baron R, Maier C, et al. Quantitative sensory testing in the German Research Network on Neuropathic Pain (DFNS): standardized protocol and reference values. Pain 2006; 123(3):231–243.
15. Gracely RH. Studies of pain in normal man. In: Melzack R, Wall PD, eds. Textbook of Pain. London: Churchill Livingstone, 1994:315–336.
16. Gracely RH, Grant MA, Giesecke T. Evoked pain measures in fibromyalgia. Best Pract Res Clin Rheumatol 2003; 17(4):593–609.
17. Forgione AG, Barber TX. A strain gauge pain stimulator. Psychophysiology 1971; 8(1):102–106.
18. Brennum J, Kjeldsen M, Jensen K, et al. Measurements of human pressure-pain thresholds on fingers and toes. Pain 1989; 38:211–217.
19. Sarlani E, Grace EG, Reynolds MA, et al. Sex differences in temporal summation of pain and aftersensations following repetitive noxious mechanical stimulation. Pain 2004; 109(1–2):115–123.
20. Kramer HH, Rolke R, Bickel A, et al. Thermal thresholds predict painfulness of diabetic neuropathies. Diabetes Care 2004; 27(10):2386–2391.
21. Curatolo M, Petersen-Felix S, Arendt-Nielsen L. Sensory assessment of regional analgesia in humans: a review of methods and applications. Anesthesiology 2000; 93(6):1517–1530.
22. Baumgartner U, Cruccu G, Iannetti GD, et al. Laser guns and hot plates. Pain 2005; 116(1–2):1–3.
23. Yeomans DC, Pirec V, Proudfit HK. Nociceptive responses to high and low rates of noxious cutaneous heating are mediated by different nociceptors in the rat: behavioral evidence. Pain 1996; 68(1):133–140.

24. Yeomans DC, Proudfit HK. Nociceptive responses to high and low rates of noxious cutaneous heating are mediated by different nociceptors in the rat: electrophysiological evidence. Pain 1996; 68(1):141–150.
25. Lotsch J, Angst MS. The mu-opioid agonist remifentanil attenuates hyperalgesia evoked by blunt and punctuated stimuli with different potency: a pharmacological evaluation of the freeze lesion in humans. Pain 2003; 102(1–2):151–161.
26. Tegeder I, Meier S, Burian M, et al. Peripheral opioid analgesia in experimental human pain models. Brain 2003; 126(pt 5):1092–1102.
27. al'Absi M, Petersen KL, Wittmers LE. Adrenocortical and hemodynamic predictors of pain perception in men and women. Pain 2002; 96(1–2):197–204.
28. Edwards RR, Kronfli T, Haythornthwaite JA, et al. Association of catastrophizing with interleukin-6 responses to acute pain. Pain 2008; 140(1):135–144.
29. Schiff E, Eisenberg E. Can quantitative sensory testing predict the outcome of epidural steroid injections in sciatica? A preliminary study. Anesth Analg 2003; 97(3):828–832.
30. Bisgaard T, Klarskov B, Rosenberg J, et al. Characteristics and prediction of early pain after laparoscopic cholecystectomy. Pain 2001; 90(3):261–269.
31. Chan CW, Dallaire M. Subjective pain sensation is linearly correlated with the flexion reflex in man. Brain Res 1989; 479:145–150.
32. Willer JC, Roby A, Le Bars D. Psychophysical and electrophysiological approaches to the pain-relieving effects of heterotopic nociceptive stimuli. Brain 1984; 107(pt 4): 1095–1112.
33. French DJ, France CR, France JL, et al. The influence of acute anxiety on assessment of nociceptive flexion reflex thresholds in healthy young adults. Pain 2005; 114(3):358–363.
34. Rhudy JL, Williams AE, McCabe KM, et al. Affective modulation of nociception at spinal and supraspinal levels. Psychophysiol 2005; 42(5):579–587.
35. Houle M, McGrath PA, Moran G, et al. The efficacy of hypnosis- and relaxation-induced analgesia on two dimensions of pain for cold pressor and electrical tooth pulp stimulation. Pain 1988; 33:241–251.
36. Moore PA, Duncan GH, Scott DS, et al. The submaximal effort tourniquet test: its use in evaluating experimental and chronic pain. Pain 1979; 6:375–382.
37. Edwards RR, Fillingim RB. Age-associated differences in responses to noxious stimuli. J Gerontol A Biol Sci Med Sci 2001; 56(3):M180–M185.
38. Segerdahl M, Karelov A. Experimentally induced ischaemic pain in healthy humans is attenuated by the adenosine receptor antagonist theophylline. Acta Physiol Scand 2004; 180(3):301–306.
39. Kosek E, Ordeberg G. Lack of pressure pain modulation by heterotopic noxious conditioning stimulation in patients with painful osteoarthritis before, but not following, surgical pain relief. Pain 2000; 88(1):69–78.
40. Campbell CM, France CR, Robinson ME, et al. Ethnic differences in diffuse noxious inhibitory controls. J Pain 2008; 9(8):759–766.
41. Fillingim RB, Maixner W, Girdler SS, et al. Ischemic but not thermal pain sensitivity varies across the menstrual cycle. Psychosom Med 1997; 59(5):512–520.
42. Fillingim RB, Maixner W, Kincaid S, et al. Pain sensitivity in patients with temporomandibular disorders: relationship to clinical and psychosocial factors. Clin J Pain 1996; 12:260–269.

43. Dirks J, Petersen KL, Rowbotham MC, et al. Gabapentin suppresses cutaneous hyperalgesia following heat-capsaicin sensitization. Anesthesiology 2002; 97(1): 102–107.

44. Frymoyer AR, Rowbotham MC, Petersen KL. Placebo-controlled comparison of a morphine/dextromethorphan combination with morphine on experimental pain and hyperalgesia in healthy volunteers. J Pain 2007; 8(1):19–25.

45. Klein T, Magerl W, Hanschmann A, et al. Antihyperalgesic and analgesic properties of the N-methyl-D-aspartate (NMDA) receptor antagonist neramexane in a human surrogate model of neurogenic hyperalgesia. Eur J Pain 2008; 12(1):17–29.

46. Zubieta JK, Smith YR, Bueller JA, et al. mu-Opioid receptor-mediated anti-nociceptive responses differ in men and women. J Neurosci 2002; 22(12):5100–5107.

47. Zubieta JK, Heitzeg MM, Smith YR, et al. COMT val158met genotype affects mu-opioid neurotransmitter responses to a pain stressor. Science 2003; 299(5610): 1240–1243.

48. Arendt-Nielsen L, Petersen-Felix S. Wind-up and neuroplasticity: is there a correlation to clinical pain? Eur J Anaesthesiol Suppl 1995; 10:1–7.

49. Melzack R, Coderre TJ, Katz J, Vaccarino AL. Central neuroplasticity and patho-logical pain. Ann N Y Acad Sci 2001; 933:157–174.

50. Herrero JF, Laird JM, Lopez-Garcia JA. Wind-up of spinal cord neurones and pain sensation: much ado about something? Prog Neurobiol 2000; 61(2):169–203.

51. Bradley LA, McKendree-Smith NL, Alarcon GS, et al. Is fibromyalgia a neurologic disease? Curr Pain Headache Rep 2002; 6(2):106–114.

52. Maixner W, Fillingim R, Sigurdsson A, et al. Sensitivity of patients with painful temporomandibular disorders to experimentally evoked pain: evidence for altered temporal summation of pain. Pain 1998; 76(1–2):71–81.

53. Sarlani E, Greenspan JD. Evidence for generalized hyperalgesia in tempor-omandibular disorders patients. Pain 2003; 102(3):221–226.

54. Sarlani E, Grace EG, Reynolds MA, et al. Evidence for up-regulated central nociceptive processing in patients with masticatory myofascial pain. J Orofac Pain 2004; 18(1):41–55.

55. Stubhaug A, Breivik H, Eide PK, et al. Mapping of punctuate hyperalgesia around a surgical incision demonstrates that ketamine is a powerful suppressor of central sen-sitization to pain following surgery. Acta Anaesthesiol Scand 1997; 41(9):1124–1132.

56. Eide PK, Stubhaug A. Relief of trigeminal neuralgia after percutaneous retrogasserian glycerol rhizolysis is dependent on normalization of abnormal temporal summation of pain, without general impairment of sensory perception. Neurosurgery 1998; 43(3): 462–472.

57. Millan MJ. Descending control of pain. Prog Neurobiol 2002; 66(6):355–474.

58. Greenspan JD, Craft RM, LeResche L, et al. Studying sex and gender differences in pain and analgesia: a consensus report. Pain 2007; 132(suppl 1):S26–S45.

59. Fillingim RB. Sex, Gender, and Pain. Seattle: IASP Press, 2000.

60. Edwards CL, Fillingim RB, Keefe F. Race, ethnicity and pain. Pain 2001; 94(2): 133–137.

61. Gatchel RJ, Turk DC. Psychosocial factors in pain. New York: Guilford Press, 1999.

62. Meagher MW, Arnau RC, Rhudy JL. Pain and emotion: effects of affective picture modulation. Psychosom Med 2001; 63(1):79–90.

63. Rhudy JL, Meagher MW. Fear and anxiety: divergent effects on human pain thresholds. Pain 2000; 84(1):65–75.

64. Zillmann D, de Wied M, King-Jablonski C, et al. Drama-induced affect and pain sensitivity. Psychosom Med 1996; 58(4):333–341.
65. Lavigne G, Zucconi M, Castronovo C, et al. Sleep arousal response to experimental thermal stimulation during sleep in human subjects free of pain and sleep problems. Pain 2000; 84(2–3):283–290.
66. Smith MT, Edwards RR, McCann UD, et al. The effects of sleep deprivation on pain inhibition and spontaneous pain in women. Sleep 2007; 30(4):494–505.
67. Lautenbacher S, Fillingim RB. Pathophysiology of Pain Perception. 1st ed. New York: Springer, 2004.
68. Woolf CJ, Max MB. Mechanism-based pain diagnosis: issues for analgesic drug development. Anesthesiology 2001; 95(1):241–249.
69. Staud R. Fibromyalgia pain: do we know the source? Curr Opin Rheumatol 2004; 16(2):157–163.
70. Granot M, Friedman M, Yarnitsky D, et al. Enhancement of the perception of systemic pain in women with vulvar vestibulitis. BJOG 2002; 109(8):863–866.
71. Wilder-Smith CH, Schindler D, Lovblad K, et al. Brain functional magnetic resonance imaging of rectal pain and activation of endogenous inhibitory mechanisms in irritable bowel syndrome patient subgroups and healthy controls. Gut 2004; 53(11): 1595–1601.
72. Ashina S, Bendtsen L, Ashina M. Pathophysiology of tension-type headache. Curr Pain Headache Rep 2005; 9(6):415–422.
73. Mogil JS, McCarson KE. Identifying pain genes: bottom-up and top-down approaches. J Pain 2000; 1(suppl 3):66–80.
74. Mogil JS, Ritchie J, Smith SB, et al. Melanocortin-1 receptor gene variants affect pain and mu-opioid analgesia in mice and humans. J Med Genet 2005; 42(7):583–587.
75. Diatchenko L, Slade GD, Nackley AG, et al. Genetic basis for individual variations in pain perception and the development of a chronic pain condition. Hum Mol Genet 2005; 14(1):135–143.
76. Kim H, Neubert JK, San MA, et al. Genetic influence on variability in human acute experimental pain sensitivity associated with gender, ethnicity and psychological temperament. Pain 2004; 109(3):488–496.
77. Lawlis GF, Achterberg J, Kenner L, et al. Ethnic and sex differences in response to clinical and induced pain in chronic spinal pain patients. Spine 1984; 9:751–754.
78. Heft MW, Gracely RH, Dubner R, et al. A validation model for verbal description scaling of human clinical pain. Pain 1980; 9(3):363–373.
79. Nikolajsen L, Ilkjaer S, Jensen TS. Relationship between mechanical sensitivity and postamputation pain: a prospective study. Eur J Pain 2000; 4(4):327–334.
80. Granot M, Lowenstein L, Yarnitsky D, et al. Postcesarean section pain prediction by preoperative experimental pain assessment. Anesthesiology 2003; 98(6):1422–1426.
81. Werner MU, Duun P, Kehlet H. Prediction of postoperative pain by preoperative nociceptive responses to heat stimulation. Anesthesiology 2004; 100(1):115–119.
82. Lundblad H, Kreicbergs A, Jansson KA. Prediction of persistent pain after total knee replacement for osteoarthritis. J Bone Joint Surg Br 2008; 90(2):166–171.
83. Rammelsberg P, LeResche L, Dworkin S, et al. Longitudinal outcome of temporomandibular disorders: a 5-year epidemiologic study of muscle disorders defined by research diagnostic criteria for temporomandibular disorders. J Orofac Pain 2003; 17(1):9–20.

84. Bernhardt O, Gesch D, Schwahn C, et al. Risk factors for headache, including TMD signs and symptoms, and their impact on quality of life. Results of the Study of Health in Pomerania (SHIP). Quintessence Int 2005; 36(1):55–64.

85. Slade GD, Diatchenko L, Bhalang K, et al. Influence of psychological factors on risk of temporomandibular disorders. J Dent Res 2007; 86(11):1120–1125.

86. Chong PS, Cros DP. Technology literature review: quantitative sensory testing. Muscle Nerve 2004; 29(5):734–747.

87. Cruccu G, Anand P, Attal N, et al. EFNS guidelines on neuropathic pain assessment. Eur J Neurol 2004; 11(3):153–162.

88. Boivie J. Central pain and the role of quantitative sensory testing (QST) in research and diagnosis. Eur J Pain 2003; 7(4):339–343.

89. Staud R, Smitherman ML. Peripheral and central sensitization in fibromyalgia: pathogenetic role. Curr Pain Headache Rep 2002; 6(4):259–266.

90. Edwards RR. Individual differences in endogenous pain modulation as a risk factor for chronic pain. Neurology 2005; 65(3):437–443.

91. Pappagallo M, Oaklander AL, Quatrano-Piacentini AL, et al. Heterogenous patterns of sensory dysfunction in postherpetic neuralgia suggest multiple pathophysiologic mechanisms. Anesthesiology 2000; 92(3):691–698.

92. Ness TJ, Powell-Boone T, Cannon R, et al. Psychophysical evidence of hypersensitivity in subjects with interstitial cystitis. J Urol 2005; 173(6):1983–1987.

93. Kleinbohl D, Holzl R, Moltner A, et al. Psychophysical measures of sensitization to tonic heat discriminate chronic pain patients. Pain 1999; 81(1–2):35–43.

94. Giesecke T, Williams DA, Harris RE, et al. Subgrouping of fibromyalgia patients on the basis of pressure-pain thresholds and psychological factors. Arthritis Rheum 2003; 48(10):2916–2922.

95. Jaaskelainen SK. The utility of clinical neurophysiological and quantitative sensory testing for trigeminal neuropathy. J Orofac Pain 2004; 18(4):355–359.

96. Jaaskelainen SK, Teerijoki-Oksa T, Forssell H. Neurophysiologic and quantitative sensory testing in the diagnosis of trigeminal neuropathy and neuropathic pain. Pain 2005; 117(3):349–357.

97. Edwards RR, Doleys DM, Lowery D, et al. Pain tolerance as a predictor of outcome following multidisciplinary treatment for chronic pain: differential effects as a function of sex. Pain 2003; 106(3):419–426.

98. Granot M, Zimmer EZ, Friedman M, et al. Association between quantitative sensory testing, treatment choice, and subsequent pain reduction in vulvar vestibulitis syndrome. J Pain 2004; 5(4):226–232.

99. Elmer GI, Peiper JO, Negus SS, et al. Genetic variation in nociception and its relationship to the potency of morphine-induced analgesia in thermal and chemical tests. Pain 1998; 75(1):129–140.

100. Mogil JS. The genetic mediation of individual differences in sensitivity to pain and its inhibition. Proc Natl Acad Sci USA 1999; 96(14):7744–7751.

101. Hsu YW, Somma J, Hung YC, et al. Predicting postoperative Pain by preoperative pressure pain assessment. Anesthesiology 2005; 103(3):613–618.

102. Edwards RR, Haythornthwaite JA, Tella P, et al. Basal heat pain thresholds predict opioid analgesia in patients with postherpetic neuralgia. Anesthesiology 2006; 104(6):1243–1248.

103. Kosek E, Ordeberg G. Abnormalities of somatosensory perception in patients with painful osteoarthritis normalize following successful treatment. Eur J Pain 2000; 4(3): 229–238.
104. Sorensen J, Bengtsson A, Ahlner J, et al. Fibromyalgia—are there different mechanisms in the processing of pain? A double blind crossover comparison of analgesic drugs. J Rheumatol 1997; 24(8):1615–1621.
105. Poitras P, Riberdy PM, Plourde V, et al. Evolution of visceral sensitivity in patients with irritable bowel syndrome. Dig Dis Sci 2002; 47(4):914–920.
106. Compton P, Charuvastra VC, Ling W. Pain intolerance in opioid-maintained former opiate addicts: effect of long-acting maintenance agent. Drug Alcohol Depend 2001; 63(2):139–146.
107. Compton P, Charuvastra VC, Kintaudi K, et al. Pain responses in methadone-maintained opioid abusers. J Pain Symptom Manage 2000; 20(4):237–245.
108. Doverty M, White JM, Somogyi AA, et al. Hyperalgesic responses in methadone maintenance patients. Pain 2001; 90(1–2):91–96.
109. Carroll IR, Angst MS, Clark JD. Management of perioperative pain in patients chronically consuming opioids. Reg AnesthPain Med 2004; 29(6):576–591.
110. Chang G, Chen L, Mao J. Opioid tolerance and hyperalgesia. Med Clin North Am 2007; 91(2):199–211.
111. Hood DD, Curry R, Eisenach JC. Intravenous remifentanil produces withdrawal hyperalgesia in volunteers with capsaicin-induced hyperalgesia. Anesth Analg 2003; 97(3):810–815.
112. Troster A, Sittl R, Singler B, et al. Modulation of remifentanil-induced analgesia and postinfusion hyperalgesia by parecoxib in humans. Anesthesiology 2006; 105(5): 1016–1023.
113. Guignard B, Bossard AE, Coste C, et al. Acute opioid tolerance: intraoperative remifentanil increases postoperative pain and morphine requirement. Anesthesiology 2000; 93(2):409–417.
114. Joly V, Richebe P, Guignard B, et al. Remifentanil-induced postoperative hyper-algesia and its prevention with small-dose ketamine. Anesthesiology 2005; 103(1): 147–155.
115. Ram KC, Eisenberg E, Haddad M, et al. Oral opioid use alters DNIC but not cold pain perception in patients with chronic pain—new perspective of opioid-induced hyperalgesia. Pain 2008; 139(2):431–438.
116. Ploghaus A, Tracey I, Gati JS, et al. Dissociating pain from its anticipation in the human brain. Science 1999; 284(5422):1979–1981.
117. Wager TD, Rilling JK, Smith EE, et al. Placebo-induced changes in FMRI in the anticipation and experience of pain. Science 2004; 303(5661):1162–1167.
118. Tracey I. Imaging pain. Br J Anaesth 2008; 101(1):32–39.
119. Giamberardino MA, Berkley KJ, Iezzi S, et al. Pain threshold variations in somatic wall tissues as a function of menstrual cycle, segmental site and tissue depth in non-dysmenorrheic women, dysmenorrheic women and men. Pain 1997; 71(2):187–197.
120. Curatolo M, Petersen-Felix S, Gerber A, et al. Remifentanil inhibits muscular more than cutaneous pain in humans. Br J Anaesth 2000; 85(4):529–532.
121. Giesecke T, Gracely RH, Grant MA, et al. Evidence of augmented central pain processing in idiopathic chronic low back pain. Arthritis Rheum 2004; 50(2):613–623.
122. Petzke F, Clauw DJ, Ambrose K, et al. Increased pain sensitivity in fibromyalgia: effects of stimulus type and mode of presentation. Pain 2003; 105(3):403–413.

123. Bajaj P, Bajaj P, Graven-Nielsen T, et al. Osteoarthritis and its association with muscle hyperalgesia: an experimental controlled study. Pain 2001; 93(2):107–114.
124. Edwards RR, Haythornthwaite JA, Sullivan MJ, et al. Catastrophizing as a mediator of sex differences in pain: differential effects for daily pain versus laboratory-induced pain. Pain 2004; 111(3):335–341.
125. Price DD, Mao J, Frenk H, et al. The $N$-methyl-D-aspartate receptor antagonist dextromethorphan selectively reduces temporal summation of second pain in man. Pain 1994; 59:165–174.
126. Eide PK. Wind-up and the NMDA receptor complex from a clinical perspective. Eur J Pain 2000; 4(1):5–15.
127. Rainville P, Feine JS, Bushnell MC, et al. A psychophysical comparison of sensory and affective responses to four modalites of experimental pain. Somatosens Mot Res 1992; 9(4):265–277.
128. Zhang X, Ashton-Miller JA, Stohler CS. A closed-loop system for maintaining constant experimental muscle pain in man. IEEE Trans Biomed Eng 1993; 40(4): 344–352.
129. Stohler CS, Kowalski CJ. Spatial and temporal summation of sensory and affective dimensions of deep somatic pain. Pain 1999; 79(2–3):165–173.
130. Coghill RC, Eisenach J. Individual differences in pain sensitivity: implications for treatment decisions. Anesthesiology 2003; 98(6):1312–1314.

# 5

# Opioid Tolerance, Dependence, and Hyperalgesia

*Penn Pain Medicine Center, University of Pennsylvania, Philadelphia,
Pennsylvania, U.S.A.*

## INTRODUCTION

Opioid tolerance, dependence, and hyperalgesia are adaptations to continued opioid use. Much is now understood about their underlying mechanisms, and there are chapters in this book outlining these mechanisms in considerable detail. This chapter is not about mechanisms, but about the interplay between opioid tolerance, dependence, and hyperalgesia, and how understanding this interplay can inform clinical practice.

Although our primary interest, as practitioners treating pain, is in pain not addiction, we have learned much by observing opioid-addicted individuals. One such observation—that after prolonged continued opioid abuse, addicts no longer experience euphoria but need to continue taking opioid to avoid dysphoria (Fig. 1)—may actually be key to understanding the adaptations that render opioids less effective as analgesics (as well as euphorics) after prolonged administration. The adaptations occur for a reason: the underlying systems, the endogenous opioid, and pain systems play a critical role in survival, and therefore they must be preserved.

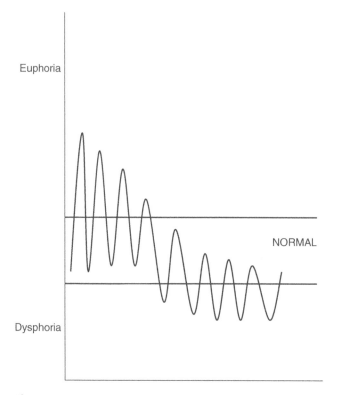

**Figure 1**  Natural history of opioid dependence. The figure illustrates the change from positive reinforcement to negative reinforcement during establishment of addiction.

## TOLERANCE AND DEPENDENCE

Tolerance can be simply defined as the need for more drugs to achieve the same effect. Yet there is nothing simple about tolerance, its mechanisms, or its manifestations. While it may be possible in clinical terms to delineate tolerance as an isolated phenomenon, as in the clinical observation that progressively higher doses are needed to achieve the same analgesic effect, in terms of process, tolerance cannot be separated from dependence. In the case of established opioid use, tolerance is necessarily bound to dependence (seen as withdrawal) because any increase in tolerance will be manifest as withdrawal (possibly subtle) unless the need for dose increase is satisfied. (Conversely, any decrease in tolerance will be manifest as overdose unless there is a dose adjustment.) In the case of early developing tolerance, it may be tolerance itself that produces the need for a higher dose, to reestablish pain relief or euphoria (positive reinforcement). Yet very quickly, dependence comes into play (negative reinforcement), and the two together drive opioid requirements, and opioid-seeking behavior should this arise

**Table 1** Reinforcing Effects of Opioids

| Positive reinforcement | Negative reinforcement |
| --- | --- |
| Euphoria, reward (mesocorticolimbic system) | Withdrawal anhedonia (let down) |
| Compensatory adaptations in regions that control somatic function, predominantly locus ceruleus. Symptomatic only on withdrawal. | Physical symptoms comprising central neurologic arousal and sleeplessness, irritability, psychomotor agitation, diarrhea, rhinorrhea, and piloerection |
| Pain relief (pain systems) | Withdrawal hyperalgesia |

*Note*: Both positive and negative effects are important drivers of opioid-seeking behavior. Negative effects predominate during established opioid use. Negative effects characterize withdrawal.
*Source*: From Refs. 1–6.

(1–6) (Table 1). The negative effects manifest in withdrawal (as determined by the level of tolerance) are likely fundamentally important in the common clinical scenario where pain relief is inadequate, yet continued opioid use is needed to avoid worsening pain and mood (withdrawal). Moreover, tolerance, and therefore dependence, does not arise as a simple continuum related to dose, but rather arises as a complex adaptation that changes in response to a wide variety of factors, including psychological and situational, and could be manifest subtly as well as grossly.

To understand how factors other than drug dose can produce symptoms related to drug use (symptoms of dependence and withdrawal, or overdose), it is necessary first to understand that tolerance is not simply a cellular or molecular adaptation, but that there is also an overlying learning process that alters the level of tolerance and the resulting symptoms. The latter has been termed *associative tolerance*, and the former *nonassociative tolerance. Associative tolerance* (which can arise in the case of all the central effects of opioids including euphoria and dysphoria, sedation, analgesia, and nausea) involves learning, and its development is linked to environmental or contextual cues (7,8). The clinical corollary is the heroin addict whose opioid requirement is reduced when placed in the situation of receiving treatment in hospital for acute pain no longer needing to procure, or conversely the chronic user placed in a stressful situation triggering an increase in tolerance and requirement. Conceivably, associative tolerance can fluctuate many times during any given day. Mechanisms of *nonassociative (pharmacological) tolerance* to opioids are better understood than those of *associative tolerance*, but even they have not been fully elucidated. Receptor changes are thought to involve internalization, recycling, desensitization, or downregulation (9–12). Many studies have implicated the $N$-methyl-D-aspartate (NMDA)-receptor in opioid tolerance, although other receptors and systems could also be involved (12–20). Processes that oppose opioid actions, for example, upregulation of cyclic adenosine monophosphate (cAMP) and CREB, have been implicated in tolerance to the hedonic effects of opioids (21). Spinal dynorphin mechanisms have been implicated in the development of opioid analgesia tolerance (22,23), while dynorphin mechanisms have also been linked to tolerance and possible dependence, leading to dysphoria (24). Several endogenous peptides oppose the analgesic effects of opioids, and are therefore termed *anti-opioid peptides.* These include vasopressin, oxytocin, nociceptin, and cholecystokinin (25–27).

A second factor in comprehending the complexity and fluctuating nature of opioid related symptoms is to understand that each component of tolerance/ dependence (i.e., reward vs. analgesia vs. side effects) is likely to arise through distinct mechanisms related to the anatomic or neuroanatomic substrate of the different effects (28–30). Thus, adaptations arise independently in the mesocorticolimic system (reward system), pain systems, and central noradrenergic nuclei (Fig. 2). This distinction is seen clinically as reward versus analgesia versus side effects arising at their own pace and magnitude. For example, during the development of addiction, tolerance to the hedonistic effects of opioids is

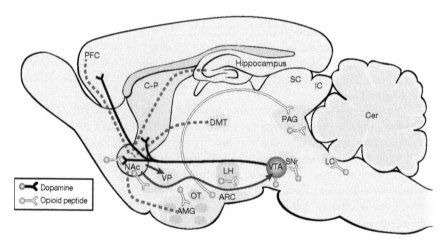

**Figure 2**   Key neural circuits of addiction. Dotted lines indicate limbic afferents to the nucleus accumbens (Nac). Black arrow lines represent efferents from the Nac thought to be involved in drug reward. ⊶ indicate projections of the mesolimbic dopamine system thought to be a critical substrate for drug reward. Dopamine neurons originate in the VTA and project to the Nac and other limbic structures, including the OT, ventral domains of the caudate-putamen (C-P), the amygdala (AMG), and the prefrontal cortex (PFC). ⊶ indicates opioid-peptide-containing neurons, which are involved in opiate, ethanol, and possibly nicotine reward. These opioid peptide systems include the local enkephalin circuits (short segments) and the hypothalamic midbrain β-endorphin circuit (long segment). *Abbreviations*: ARC, arcuate nucleus; Cer, cerebellum; DMT, dorsomedial thalamus; IC, inferior colliculus; LC, locus coeruleus; LH, lateral hypothalamus; PAG, peraqueductal grey; SC, superior colliculus; SNr, substantia nigra pars reticulata; VP, ventral pallidum; VTA, ventral tegmental area; OT, olfactory tubercle. *Source*: Adapted from Ref. 21.

marked, to the extent that tolerance, and the need to take increasing doses to achieve intoxication or the desired effect, characterizes opioid addiction (as well as addiction to several other substances) (31). In contrast, analgesic tolerance is less obvious. Some clinicians even argue that since there may be stable analgesia after initial titration, with no need for dose escalation, there is no pharmacological (physiological) tolerance to the analgesic effects of opioids. Yet the need for escalating doses in the absence of disease progression is also observed (32,33), as is the need for higher than usual doses when acute pain arises in patients receiving chronic opioid treatment (34–38). Others argue, then, that there must be a pharmacological mechanism for opioid analgesic tolerance. Supporting this argument, animal studies of reflex pain responses (absence of influence from higher centers) show marked analgesic tolerance (39–41) and classical studies in humans also show the effect (42). Moreover, returning to the concept that opioid-induced adaptations involve psychological (associative or learned) effects as well as direct drug effects (pharmacological component), and occur at multiple locations (28,40,43), it would seem unlikely that pain itself could be completely isolated from the other effects, at least in terms of fluctuations in dose-related symptoms.

Side effects arise predominantly through opioid effects at central nuclei such as the respiratory center (respiratory depression) and chemoreceptor trigger zone (nausea). Likewise, tolerance to each side effect must arise through different mechanisms at different central locations. Because bowel effects are largely mediated directly through receptors on the bowel itself, and are less affected by the type of neuroadaptations that arise in the CNS, there is generally no tolerance to the bowel slowing effects of opioids.

## WITHDRAWAL

*Dependence* is the term used to describe a state of continued habitual drug use that will result in a withdrawal syndrome when the drug is withdrawn. The word *withdrawal* suggests that drug must actually be withdrawn to induce symptoms. However, in line with the previous discussion about the link between tolerance and dependence, and the fluctuating nature of these, it is feasible that withdrawal symptoms may arise even in the absence of drug withdrawal. Dependence could therefore be seen as a state in which the individual is liable to withdrawal symptoms because of habitual drug use, even in the absence of drug withdrawal.

Because addicts in withdrawal manifest a characteristic constellation of largely physical symptoms, *withdrawal* is often described as physical syndrome, ignoring the psychological component and the pain manifestations. This is true in texts on addiction and pain, in guidelines, and in addiction criteria. One of the great difficulties we face in understanding dependence during opioid treatment of pain is just this: while the manifestations of dependence in addicts may include many of the same characteristics and those in pain patients, their relative dominance is very different. Thus, the addict in withdrawal exhibits a characteristic opioid withdrawal syndrome with central neurologic arousal and sleeplessness, irritability, psychomotor agitation, diarrhea, rhinorrhea, and piloerection. The pain patient, on the other hand, is more likely to simply experience a general feeling of malaise or being let down (withdrawal anhedonia), possibly a worsening of pain or an increase in pain sensitivity (withdrawal hyperalgesia), and no overt physical symptoms. This state in pain patients could be thought of as a subthreshold withdrawal. This difference between withdrawal states in addicts and pain patients can be explained partly by the fact that doses and dose fluctuations in pain patients are typically much smaller than in addicts.

Physical dependence is the manifestation of compensatory adaptations in brain regions that control somatic functions: in the case of opioids, an important region affected is the noradrenergic nucleus, the locus coeruleus (Fig. 2) (44,45). The physical symptoms of opioid withdrawal appear to result, at least in part, from an upregulation of cAMP and noradrenergic mechanisms in the locus coeruleus or other brain regions (21,29). Hyperalgesia is often described as a component of the physical withdrawal syndrome, but may not actually be related to noradrenergic mechanisms (46).

While withdrawal hyperalgesia has long been recognized as part of the constellation of symptoms of the opioid withdrawal syndrome (46–48), more recently the phenomenon of opioid-induced hyperalgesia during opioid treatment (not just during withdrawal) is recognized as clinically important (37,49–56). Treatment-related opioid hyperalgesia was first observed in methadone-maintained addicts (52,57–59), but more recently clinical situations have arisen where the phenomenon seems to interfere with the success of opioid pain therapy. For example, patients treated with potent or high-dose opioid infusions display hyperalgesia with characteristic skin sensitivity (allodynia), which resolves once the infusion is weaned (60–62). Although none are fully elucidated, there are many proposed mechanisms for opioid-induced hyperalgesia, described in other chapters of this book. One intriguing possibility is that even though manifest during opioid administration and not during opioid withdrawal, withdrawal (or subtle withdrawal) may account, at least in part, for the phenomenon. The recent identification of a top-down system of reciprocal control of pain operating through two distinct neuronal subpopulations ("off" cells and "on" cells), in turn inhibited or disinhibited by opioids, helps to explain how opioid drugs can either relieve or worsen pain depending on behavioral state (63). For example, these subtypes exhibit reciprocal changes in firing just before a withdrawal reflex, which can be demonstrated experimentally during the presence of a predator. Hyperalgesia (enhancing protective reflexes) is as necessary to recovery and survival as is analgesia (stress induced analgesia), so it is not difficult to see why, recognizing that the endogenous pain and opioid systems are critical to survival, hyperalgesia would be part of the spectrum of opioid effects.

*Psychological dependence* is manifest as the psychological component of withdrawal and must be distinguished from *physical dependence*. Psychological dependence comprises both unpleasant emotional effects (withdrawal anhedonia and dysphoria) (3,4,28,30) and motivational effects (craving during withdrawal), the latter being partly mediated by physical withdrawal. Mechanisms for the psychological dependence likely arise in the mesocorticolimbic system, the so-called reward center (Fig. 2). The symptoms of withdrawal, whether physical or psychological, are powerful drivers of opioid-seeking behavior and apparent opioid tolerance (3,4,45,64). Thus, the symptoms that accompany withdrawal and drive up opioid doses can easily be interpreted as inadequacy of pain relief. These effects might be particularly noticed after prolonged opioid therapy, when, as is seen in the parallel addiction population, the positive reinforcing effects of opioids diminish, so opioid seeking becomes largely driven by the negative reinforcing effects of withdrawal (1–6). Moreover, since psychological symptoms associated with withdrawal (e.g., dysphoria and depression) can worsen the underlying pain syndrome (65–69), withdrawal may actually drive up measured pain scores.

## DEFINITIONS

This chapter argues that withdrawal phenomena are important to the clinical picture of diminishing efficacy from prolonged continuous opioids pain therapy, where higher doses leave pain unabated, yet with lower doses pain reemerges. It argues that tolerance and dependence, once established during continued use, cannot be delineated as independent phenomena, and that dependence in opioid-treated pain patients is a different state to that in addicts in its clinical characteristics and its underlying mechanisms. Our core difficulty has been to understand opioid dependence in the context of opioid treatment of pain, and part of this difficulty has been that definitions of dependence are at best inadequate, and at worst misleading and confusing.

The story starts early in the 20th century when both clinicians and scientists struggled to understand and define addiction. Definitions became necessary to advance the addiction field in terms of both treatment and understanding basic mechanisms. Although there have been many iterations, the present-day DSM-IV criteria for "substance dependence" (the term chosen for what is understood in general parlance as "drug addiction") define clear criteria for the clinical picture of drug addiction, and these criteria are generally established and accepted (Table 2) (31). Here, there are seven addiction criteria, five of which are behavioral, the other two being tolerance and physical dependence. Since three or more criteria must be met for a diagnosis of substance dependence, at least one behavioral criterion must be present, but tolerance and physical dependence are not necessarily present. The fact that these definitions are widely accepted is an indication that for most purposes, and in the case of addiction, they are useful. However, once opioid treatment of chronic

**Table 2** DSM-IV Substance Dependence Criteria

Addiction (termed *substance dependence* by the American Psychiatric Association) is defined as a maladaptive pattern of substance use, leading to clinically significant impairment or distress, as manifested by three (or more) of the following, occurring at any time in the same 12-month period:

1. Tolerance, as defined by either of the following:

    (a) A need for markedly increased amount of the substance to achieve intoxication or the desired effect

    *or*

    (b) markedly diminished effect with continued use of the same amount of the substance.

2. Withdrawal, as manifested by either of the following:

    (a) The characteristic withdrawal syndrome for the substance

    *or*

    (b) the same (or closely related) substance is taken to relieve or avoid withdrawal symptoms.

3. The substance is often taken in larger amounts or over a longer period than intended.
4. There is a persistent desire or unsuccessful efforts to cut down or control substance use.
5. A great deal of time is spent in activities necessary to obtain the substance, use the substance, or recover from its effects.
6. Important social, occupational, or recreational activities are given up or reduced because of substance use.
7. The substance use is continued despite the knowledge of having a persistent physical or psychological problem that is likely to have been caused or exacerbated by the substance.

*Source*: From Ref. 31.

pain became more widespread at the end of the 20th century, it was quickly recognized by those involved in this therapy that the DSM and other standard addiction criteria (70,71) were misleading when applied to pain patients. This was partly because drug was prescribed not procured (thus markedly altering the behaviors around drug use), and, perhaps more importantly, because dependence was an inevitable accompaniment to treatment, and not necessarily an indication of addiction. Because of this difficulty, a group of pain physicians and addiction specialists devised a new set of definitions for use in pain patients outlined in Table 3 (72). Here tolerance, physical dependence, and addiction are presented as three separate phenomena. These consensus definitions have never been fully accepted, and in fact they are presently under review because they, despite their intention, are also problematic and misleading in terms of interpreting the manifestations of chronic drug use in opioid-treated pain patients. What is suggested by the consensus definitions is that (*i*) tolerance and dependence arise in isolation, (*ii*) dependence is simply a physical phenomenon, and (*iii*) the psychological component of dependence (anhenonia) and associated behaviors

**Table 3** Consensus Definitions Related to the Use of Opioids for the Treatment of Pain

1. Tolerance
   Tolerance is a state of adaptation in which exposure to a drug induces changes that result in a diminution of one or more of the drug's effects over time.
2. Physical dependence
   Physical dependence is a state of adaptation that is manifested by a drug class–specific withdrawal syndrome that can be produced by abrupt cessation, rapid dose reduction, decreasing blood level of the drug, and/or administration of an antagonist.
3. Addiction
   Addiction is a primary, chronic, neurobiologic disease, with genetic, psychosocial, and environmental factors influencing its development and manifestations. It is characterized by behaviors that include one or more of the following: impaired control over drug use, compulsive use, continued use despite harm, and craving.

*Source*: From Ref. 72.

(opioid seeking) arise only in the case of addiction. Perhaps most misleading has been the use of these definitions to teach that in opioid-treated pain patients, while physical dependence may be inevitable, the psychological component arises only in the extreme case of addiction.

To summarize, the DSM definitions suggest that all dependence is addiction, while the consensus definitions suggest that all dependence is physical. Neither is true during opioid treatment of pain, and this is where new definitions for use in pain patients are needed to foster a better understanding, particularly of the phenomenon of dependence as an adaptation to continuous opioid therapy that could affect pain relief, well-being, mood, and behavior, but is not necessarily addiction, or simply physical (73).

## CONCLUSION

If one considers that endogenous opioid systems have an important phylogenetic role, that these systems allow the animal to tolerate pain, withdraw when appropriate, fight when appropriate, repeat aversive events when appropriate, and ultimately drive behaviors that are advantageous, it is not surprising that they manifest a spectrum of effects. Thus, the opioid system does not simply produce analgesia and reward, but rather a complex balance between analgesia and hyperalgesia, euphoria and dysphoria, which alters according to circumstance and need. We use opioid drugs to treat pain because experience has taught that these mimickers of endogenous opioids provide excellent analgesia. It is not surprising, though, that under some circumstances, we might see hyperalgesia and not analgesia. The classic observation was that this occurred during withdrawal from opioids, yet more recently it seems that this is not the only circumstance in which we see it. As more opioids are used clinically, for prolonged treatment of chronic and cancer pain, and in very large doses for stress suppression during invasive surgery and prolonged intensive care, the existence of hyperalgesia as a phenomenon that interferes with opioid analgesic efficacy has emerged.

Progress is being made toward understanding whether induced hyper-algesia is related to dose, route of administration, duration, timing (continuous versus intermittent), drug choice, or underlying genetic factors. But whether or not a treatment manipulation can be pinpointed to avoid interference by hyperalgesia, it must be accepted that hyperalgesia is part of the spectrum of opioid effects, and that the balance between analgesia and hyperalgesia is likely to be altered by exogenous opioid administration. All the adaptations that are seen, whether tolerance, dependence, or hyperalgesia, make sense in terms of preserving an underlying system that exists for survival. The message in terms of clinical practice is that dependence is an inevitable consequence of continued opioid use, it can be manifest as a myriad of psychological and physical effects, including hyperalgesia, and it may seriously compromise opioid efficacy. When opioid treatment is not working, less may be better than more.

## REFERENCES

1. Robinson TE, Berridge KC. Incentive-sensitization and addiction. Addiction 2001; 96:103–114.
2. Robinson TE, Berridge KC. Addiction. Annu Rev Psychol 2003; 54:25–53.
3. Koob GF, Le Moal M. Drug abuse: hedonic homeostatic dysregulation. Science 1997; 278:52–58.
4. Koob GF, Le Moal M. Drug addiction, dysregulation of reward, and allostasis. Neuropsychopharmacology 2001; 24:97–129.
5. Gardner EL. The neurobiology and genetics of addiction: implications of the reward deficiency syndrome for therapeutic strategies in chemical dependency. In: Elster J, ed. Addiction: Entries and Exits. New York: Russell Sage Foundation, 1999:57–119.
6. Gardner EL. Brain-reward mechanisms. In: Lowinson JH, Ruiz P, Milman RB, et al., eds. Substance Abuse: A Comprehensive Textbook. Philadelphia: Lippincott Williams & Wilkins, 2005:48–97.
7. Mitchell JM, Basbaum AI, Fields HL. A locus and mechanism of action for asso-ciative morphine tolerance. Nat Neurosci 2000; 3:47–53.
8. Grisel JE, Watkins LR, Maier SF. Associative and non-associative mechanisms of morphine analgesic tolerance are neurochemically distinct in the rat spinal cord. Psychopharmacology (Berlin) 1996; 128:248–255.
9. Bohn LM, Gainetdinov RR, Lin FT, et al. Mu-opioid receptor desensitization by beta-arrestin-2 determines morphine tolerance but not dependence. Nature 2000; 408:720–723.
10. Taylor DA, Fleming WW. Unifying perspectives of the mechanisms underlying the development of tolerance and physical dependence to opioids. J Pharmacol Exp Ther 2001; 297:11–18.
11. Watts VJ. Molecular mechanisms for heterologous sensitization of adenylate cyclase. J Pharmacol Exp Ther 2002; 302:1–7.

12. He L, Whistler JL. An opiate cocktail that reduces morphine tolerance and dependence. Curr Biol 2005; 15:1028–1033.
13. Trujillo KA. Are NMDA receptors involved in opiate-induced neural and behavioral plasticity? A review of preclinical studies. Psychopharmacology (Berlin) 2000; 151:121–141.
14. Nitsche JF, Schuller AG, King MA, et al. Genetic dissociation of opiate tolerance and physical dependence in delta-opioid receptor-1 and preproenkephalin knock-out mice. J Neurosci 2002; 22:10906–10913.
15. Caspi A, Sugden K, Moffitt TE, et al. Influence of life stress on depression: moderation by a polymorphism in the 5-HTT gene [see comment]. Science 2003; 301:386–389.
16. Raith K, Hochhaus G. Drugs used in the treatment of opioid tolerance and physical dependence: a review. Int J Clin Pharmacol Ther 2004; 42:191–203.
17. Lim G, Wang S, Zeng Q, et al. Spinal glucocorticoid receptors contribute to the development of morphine tolerance in rats. Anesthesiology 2005; 102:832–837.
18. Lim G, Wang S, Zeng Q, et al. Evidence for a long-term influence on morphine tolerance after previous morphine exposure: role of neuronal glucocorticoid receptors. Pain 2005; 114:81–92.
19. Lim G, Wang S, Zeng Q, et al. Expression of spinal NMDA receptor and PKCgamma after chronic morphine is regulated by spinal glucocorticoid receptor. J Neurosci 2005; 25:11145–11154.
20. Zhao M, Joo DT. Enhancement of spinal $N$-methyl-D-aspartate receptor function by remifentanil action at delta-opioid receptors as a mechanism for acute opioid-induced hyperalgesia or tolerance. Anesthesiology 2008; 109:308–317.
21. Nestler EJ. Molecular mechanisms of drug addiction. Neuropharmacology 2004; 47(suppl. 1):24–32.
22. Vanderah TW, Gardell LR, Burgess SE, et al. Dynorphin promotes abnormal pain and spinal opioid antinociceptive tolerance. J Neurosci 2000; 20:7074–7079.
23. Vanderah TW, Ossipov MH, Lai J, et al. Mechanisms of opioid-induced pain and antinociceptive tolerance: descending facilitation and spinal dynorphin. Pain 2001; 92:5–9.
24. Carlezon W, Duman R, Nestler EJ. The many faces of CREB. Trends Neurosci 2005; 28:436–445.
25. Cesselin F. Opioid and anti-opioid peptides. Fundam Clin Pharmacol 1995; 9: 409–433.
26. Wiesenfeld-Hallin Z, Xu XJ. Neuropeptides in neuropathic and inflammatory pain with special emphasis on cholecystokinin and galanin. Eur J Pharmacol 2001; 429:49–59.
27. Xu XJ, Colpaert F, Wiesenfeld-Hallin Z. Opioid hyperalgesia and tolerance versus 5-HT1A receptor-mediated inverse tolerance. Trends Pharmacol Sci 2003; 24:634–639.
28. Koob GF, Maldonado R, Stinus L. Neural substrates of opiate withdrawal. Trends Neurosci 1992; 15:186–191.
29. Nestler EJ, Aghajanian GK. Molecular and cellular basis of addiction. Science 1997; 278:58–63.
30. Hyman SE, Malenka RC, Nestler EJ. Neural mechanisms of addiction: the role of reward-related learning and memory. Annu Rev Neurosci 2006; 29:565–598.
31. American Psychiatric Association. Diagnostic and Statistical Manual of Mental Disorders. 4th ed. Washington, DC: American Psychiatric Association, 1994.

32. Bruera E, Brenneis C, Michaud M, et al. Use of the subcutaneous route for the administration of narcotics in patients with cancer pain. Cancer 1988; 62:407–411.
33. Mercadante S, Bruera E. Opioid switching: a systematic and critical review. Cancer Treat Rev 2006; 32:304–315.
34. de Leon-Casasola OA, Myers DP, Donaparthi S, et al. A comparison of postoperative epidural analgesia between patients with chronic cancer taking high doses of oral opioids versus opioid-naive patients. Anesth Analg 1993; 76:302–307.
35. Rapp SE, Ready LB, Nessly ML. Acute pain management in patients with prior opioid consumption: a case-controlled retrospective review. Pain 1995; 61:195–201.
36. Mitra S, Sinatra RS. Perioperative management of acute pain in the opioid-dependent patient. Anesthesiology 2004; 101:212–227.
37. Angst MS, Clark JD. Opioid-induced hyperalgesia: a qualitative systematic review. Anesthesiology 2006; 104:570–587.
38. Wilder-Smith OH, Arendt-Nielsen L. Postoperative hyperalgesia: its clinical importance and relevance. Anesthesiology 2006; 104:601–607.
39. Yu W, Hao JX, Xu XJ, et al. The development of morphine tolerance and dependence in rats with chronic pain. Brain Res 1997; 756:141–146.
40. South SM, Smith MT. Analgesic tolerance to opioids. Pain Clin Updates IASP Press 2001; 9:1–4.
41. Bailey CP, Connor M. Opioids: cellular mechanisms of tolerance and physical dependence. Curr Opin Pharmacol 2005; 5:60–68.
42. McQuay H. Opioids in pain management. Lancet 1999; 353:2229–2232.
43. von Zastrow M. A cell biologist's perspective on physiological adaptation to opiate drugs. Neuropharmacology 2004; 47(suppl. 1):286–292.
44. Hyman SE. Dispelling the myths about addiction. Washington: Institute of Medicine National Academy of Sciences Press, 1997:44–46.
45. Cami J, Farre M. Drug addiction. N Engl J Med 2003; 349:975–986.
46. Compton P, Athanasos P, Elashoff D. Withdrawal hyperalgesia after acute opioid physical dependence in nonaddicted humans: a preliminary study. J Pain 2003; 4:511–519.
47. Alford DP, Compton P, Samet JH. Acute pain management for patients receiving maintenance methadone or buprenorphine therapy. Ann Intern Med 2006; 144:127–134.
48. Compton P, Darakjian JM, Miotto K. Screening for addiction in patients with chronic pain with "problematic" substance use: evaluation of a pilot assessment tool. J Pain Symptom Manage 1998; 16:355–363.
49. Brodner RA, Taub A. Chronic pain exacerbated by long-term narcotic use in patients with non-malignant disease: clinical syndrome and treatment. Mt Sinai J Med 1978; 45:233–237.
50. Taylor CB, Zlutnick SI, Corley MJ, et al. The effects of detoxification, relaxation and brief supportive therapy on chronic pain. Pain 1980; 8:319–329.
51. Savage SR. Long-term opioid therapy: assessment of consequences and risks. J Pain Symptom Manage 1996; 11:274–286.
52. Compton MA. Cold-pressor pain tolerance in opiate and cocaine abusers: correlates of drug type and use status. J Pain Symptom Manage 1994; 9:462–473.
53. Chu LF, Clark DJ, Angst MS. Opioid tolerance and hyperalgesia in chronic pain patients after one month of oral morphine therapy: a preliminary prospective study. J Pain 2006; 7:43–48.

54. Devulder J. Hyperalgesia induced by high-dose intrathecal sufentanil in neuropathic pain. J Neurosurg Anesthesiol 1997; 9:146–148.
55. Vorobeychik Y, Chen L, Bush MC, et al. Improved opioid analgesic effect following opioid dose reduction. Pain Med 2008; 9:724–727.
56. Chu LF, Angst MS, Clark D. Opioid-induced hyperalgesia in humans: molecular mechanisms and clinical considerations. Clin J Pain 2008; 24:479–496.
57. Doverty M, White JM, Somogyi AA, et al. Hyperalgesic responses in methadone maintenance patients [see comment]. Pain 2001; 90:91–96.
58. Jamison RN, Kauffman J, Katz NP. Characteristics of methadone maintenance patients with chronic pain. J Pain Sympt Manage 2000; 19:53–62.
59. Rosenblum A, Joseph H, Fong C, et al. Prevalence and characteristics of chronic pain among chemically dependent patients in methadone maintenance and residential treatment facilities. JAMA 2003; 289:2370–2378.
60. Angst MS, Koppert W, Pahl I, et al. Short-term infusion of the mu-opioid agonist remifentanil in humans causes hyperalgesia during withdrawal. Pain 2003; 106:49–57.
61. Hood DD, Curry R, Eisenach JC. Intravenous remifentanil produces withdrawal hyperalgesia in volunteers with capsaicin-induced hyperalgesia. Anesth Analg 2003; 97:810–815.
62. Guignard B, Bossard AE, Coste C, et al. Acute opioid tolerance: intraoperative remifentanil increases postoperative pain and morphine requirement. Anesthesiology 2000; 93:409–417.
63. Fields H. State-dependent opioid control of pain. Nat Rev Neurosci 2004; 5:565–575.
64. Ballantyne JC, Mao J. Opioid therapy for chronic pain. N Engl J Med 2003; 349:1943–1953.
65. Fishbain D, Cutler R, Rosomoff HL, et al. Chronic pain-associated depression: antecedent or consequence of chronic pain? A review. Clin J Pain 1997; 113:116–137.
66. Dersh J, Polatin PB, Gatchell RJ. Chronic pain and psychopathology: research finding and theoretical considerations. Psychosom Med 2002; 64:773–786.
67. McWilliams L, Goodwin R, Cox B. Depression and anxiety associated with three pain conditions: results from a nationally representative sample. Pain 2004; 111:77–83.
68. Wasan AD, Davar G, Jamison R. The association between negative affect and opioid analgesia in patients with discogenic low back pain. Pain 2005; 117:450–461.
69. Sullivan MD, Edlund MJ, Zhang L, et al. Association between mental health disorders, problem drug use, and regular prescription opioid use. Arch Intern Med 2006; 166:2087–2093.
70. World Health Organization. The ICD-10 Classification of Mental and Behavioral Disorders: Clinical Descriptions and Diagnostic Guidelines. Geneva, Switzerland: WHO, 1992.
71. WHO Expert Committee on Drug Dependence. 30th report. Geneva, Switzerland: WHO, 1998.
72. Heit HA. Addiction, physical dependence, and tolerance: precise definitions to help clinicians evaluate and treat chronic pain patients (review). J Pain Palliat Care Pharmacother 2003; 17:15–29.
73. Ballantyne JC, LaForge SL. Opioid dependence and addiction in opioid-treated pain patients. Pain 2007; 129:235–255.

## 6

# Challenging Clinical Issues on the Interaction Between Addiction and Hyperalgesia

**Walter Ling**

*Department of Psychiatry and Biobehavioral Sciences, David Geffen School of Medicine, University of California at Los Angeles, Los Angeles, California, U.S.A.*

**Peggy Compton**

*School of Nursing, University of California at Los Angeles, Los Angeles, California, U.S.A.*

## INTRODUCTION

### First Observations and History

If addiction and the relief of suffering are partners in an uneasy marriage where opiates are concerned, then opioid-induced hyperalgesia (OIH) is the mother-in-law whose role in the union may be ambiguous but whose presence is never in doubt. During the Civil War, Silas Weir Mitchell, a surgeon who, with William Alexander Hammond, is sometimes known as the Father of American Neurology, suffered a bullet wound to his neck necessitating several months of morphine use for pain relief. The following description of his experience of OIH remains one of the best to date.

> If any man wants to learn sympathetic charity, let him keep pain subdued for six months by morphia and then make the experiment of giving up the drug. By this time he will have become irritable, nervous and cowardly.

The nerves, muffled, so to speak, by narcotics will have grown to be not less sensitive but acutely, abnormally capable of feeling pain and of feeling as pain a multitude of things not usually competent to cause it (1).

So many Civil War soldiers were said to be "addicted" to morphine that it became known as the "soldier's disease." As we now understand it, however, it is unclear whether these soldiers were true addicts or simply dependent on opiates physically.

About the same time, in his essay describing his clinical observations on patients injecting morphine on a daily basis, physician and author Albutt (2) asked, "Does morphia tend to encourage the very pain it pretends to relieve?" He continued, "I have much reason to suspect that a reliance upon hypodermic morphia only ended in a curious state of *perpetuated pain*" (p. 329). Although poorly explored in the subsequent clinical research, questions about the pain responses of addicted patients again arose with the institution of methadone maintenance in the 1960s, culminating the in current understanding of what is described as opioid-OIH, or diminished tolerance for pain following opioid administration in persons exposed to opioids on a regular basis (for reviews, see Refs. 3–6).

## CLINICAL EVIDENCE OF HYPERALGESIA IN OPIOID ADDICTS

Hypothesizing over 40 years ago that opioid addicts self-medicate to deal with "an abnormally low tolerance for painful stimuli" (p. 224), Martin and Inglis (7) found significantly increased sensitivity to cold pressor (CP) pain in an incarcerated population of women described as "known narcotic addicts," in comparison to matched "nonaddict" controls. Subsequently, Ho and Dole (8) found that drug-free ex-addicts and methadone-maintained former heroin addicts were significantly more sensitive to pain induced by CP pain compared to drug-free controls. Although, since last opioid use and the presence of opioid withdrawal symptoms were not reported in these early trials, the magnitude of the relationships was impressive and suggested a phenomenon of clinical significance.

Most of what is known about the pain responses of opioid addicts has been learned from patients enrolled in methadone maintenance (MM) for the treatment of opioid addiction. These are individuals for whom opioid dosing, illicit drug use, and withdrawal symptoms are relatively well controlled, providing research subjects who are relatively reliable participants and informants (as compared to street addicts). Integration of these studies is complicated by the use of different pain induction techniques [electrical stimulation (ES), mechanical pressure (MP), cold pressor (CP)], the measurement of pain *threshold* versus pain *tolerance*, and the effects of methadone blood level (peak vs. trough) on pain responses.

Across all pain stimuli, pain *threshold* (the point at which a non-nociceptive stimulus becomes painful) has most consistently been shown to be either no different or significantly lower for MM patients in comparison with matched normal controls, under both methadone peak and trough conditions (9–14). Within-group data show that methadone dosing either had no effect on, or improved threshold for both CP and ES pain (12,15). In this, pain thresholds tend to be relatively constant across individuals in general, it is possible that the absolute detection of pain is less reflective of hyperalgesia, which is essentially a subjective assessment.

Differences between MM and controls have been more robust on measures of pain *tolerance* (the point at which the subject reports that the pain can no longer be tolerated), which conceptually may be a better representation of a hyperalgesic state. Doverty et al. show decreased tolerance for ES pain under both peak and trough methadone conditions (12,16). With respect to CP pain, significantly diminished tolerance has been consistently demonstrated in MM patients' in comparison with both matched drug-free addicts (9) and matched controls (10–13,16–17), regardless of methadone blood levels. With respect to perceived pain severity, using visual analogue scales, Schall et al. (14) found no difference between MM and control subjects in their perception of MP, while Pud et al. (17) found a significantly increased rating of CP pain in the former. When evaluated within subjects, this work indicates a significant analgesic effect for methadone on CP, ES, and MP tolerance two to four hours postdose, and this effect correlates with peak methadone blood levels (13–14).

These cross-sectional data show that MM patients are reliably intolerant of experimental pain, and are on average, between 42% and 76% less tolerant of CP pain than are normal controls matched on age, gender, and ethnicity. With appreciable (albeit trough) methadone blood levels, these patients not only appreciate *no* underlying analgesic effect from daily, high dose administration of methadone, but they also actually present a case for the *antianalgesic* (hyperalgesic) effects of chronic methadone therapy. Pilot data suggest that degree of CP hyperalgesia varies with the intrinsic activity of the opioid maintenance agent, such that patients maintained on the partial agonist buprenorphine are less hyperalgesic than those maintained on the full agonist methadone (11). Daily methadone dose, however, is not significantly related to the degree of hyperalgesia noted (9,10,16).

## Why are Addicts Hyperalgesic?

### They are Born That Way

One explanation for diminished pain tolerance in opioid-addicted patients is that they are pain sensitive by nature. Well-recognized individual differences in pain tolerance and opioid response have long been appreciated at the clinical level, and the genetic factors that underlie these differences are increasingly elucidated. An analysis of the preclinical literature (most notably from the laboratories of Mogil et al. (18,19) and Elmer and colleagues (20–22) reveals that those murine strains that demonstrate poor tolerance to pain are the same as those who are unlikely to appreciate good opioid analgesia. In addition, these pain-intolerant animals are likely to find opioids highly rewarding or "addicting" (Table 1), thus suggesting a positive relationship between pain sensitivity and opioid addiction.

**Table 1**  Pain and Opioid Responses in Murine Strains

| | BALB/c (common inbred) | CXBH (recombinant inbred) | C57 (common inbred) | CXBK (recombinant inbred) |
|---|---|---|---|---|
| Pain tolerance | ↑ (22) | ↑ (22) | ↓ (22) | ↓ (22) |
| Analgesic response | ↑ (21, 23–28) | ↑ (20, 21, 23) | ↓ (20, 21, 24–27, 29, 30) | ↓ (18, 20, 21, 23, 31, 32) |
| Reinforcement/ reward responses | ↓ (21, 24) | ↓ (21) | ↑ (21, 24, 33, 34) | ↑ (21) |
| Thermal hyperalgesia | ↓ (35) | | ↑ (35) | |
| Opioid receptor binding | ↑ (21) | ↑ (18, 21) | ± (21, 36) | ↓ (18, 21, 37, 38) |

With the advent of molecular genetics, investigators in both the pain and substance abuse fields quickly began focusing on polymorphisms in the μ-opioid gene receptor (OPRM) as candidate genes underlying phenotypes for (*i*) pain sensitivity (39–43); (*ii*) opioid analgesic response (44–46); and (*iii*) addiction (47–49). Similarly, Kest et al. reported murine strain differences in the development of opioid tolerance (50) and withdrawal severity (50,51). Probably the best characterized candidate gene is the single nucleotide polymorphism A118G of the OPRM, such that human subjects with the variant allele have been shown to require almost twice as high a plasma level of morphine to achieve the analgesic response of those with the nonmutated allele (52). Other genes that have been linked to pain and opioid responses include those that code for the delta opioid receptor (53), the capsaicin sensing vanilloid receptor (53–55), the neurotransmitter enzyme catechol-*o*-methyl transferase (53), and the melanocortin-1 receptor (56).

Genetic differences, in response to opioids, portend individual variability in the propensity to develop hyperalgesia. Building upon preliminary evidence for genetic differences in hyperalgesia development in response to opioid administration (57), Liang et al. (35) evaluated 15 different strains of mice for the development of thermal hyperalgesia after four days of morphine pretreatment, and found significant variation among strains. Percent reduction in nociceptive thresholds ranged from 29% (129/SvlmJ strain) to 89% (MRL/Mpj strain) in these experiments, and interestingly, a strain found to be relatively pain intolerant (C57BL/6J) in previous work (Table 1) also developed a high degree of hyperalgesia (87.3%) following chronic morphine administration. Suggesting a non-opioid-mediated mechanism for this hyperalgesia, haplotypic genetic analyses revealed that differential expression of the $\beta_2$-adrenergic receptor gene best explained strain-related differences in the development of thermal hyperalgesia following morphine administration (35), which may be related to opioid-induced upregulation of the receptor in the central and peripheral nervous systems.

If pain intolerance is, in fact, a genetically determined trait, addicted persons should evidence poor pain tolerance in comparison to controls, regardless of whether they currently are using drugs or are in drug-free recovery. With respect to pain *thresholds*, however, this does not appear to be the case. A series of studies by Liebmann et al. (58–60) provide evidence that drug-free opioid addicts are less sensitive to pain than are controls. These investigators report increased CP pain thresholds in ex-opioid addicts as compared to controls, a finding more recently confirmed by Prosser et al. (61) using quantitative sensory testing. Further, Lehofer and colleagues (60) reported that, using guided subjective recall, ex-opioid addicts rated themselves as less sensitive to pain than did normal controls, both when actively using opioids and when opioid-free. A genetic influence on pain *tolerance* is suggested by the data of Pud et al. (17) who found significant hyperalgesia to the CP in opioid addicts as compared to matched controls, an effect which persisted over of 28 days of opioid abstinence. Identified was a distinct subgroup of pain-intolerant ex-opioid addicts who were almost three times as likely to relapse within two years of treatment entry as were pain-tolerant ex-addicts (59). Opioid addicts with poor pain tolerance may suffer a more severe form of addiction or have difficulty tolerating the discomfort (pain) inherent in detoxification and early abstinence.

At this time, trait responses to opioids cannot be ruled out in the variable development of hyperalgesia, such that the expression of opioid-relevant genes may, in fact, play a role in propensity for opioid addiction and pain responses. But undoubtedly, the phenotypic expression of these opioid responses is both polygenetic and multifactorial, with environmental and learned effects often predominant in the pain responses of addicts in the clinical setting.

### They Are in Withdrawal

Hyperalgesia, or hypersensitivity to noxious stimuli, has long been identified as an important symptom of the opioid withdrawal syndrome. In preclinical models, when opioid agonist administration is either abruptly terminated (62–67) or reversed by an antagonist (68–73), hyperalgesia is reliably demonstrated to thermal (tail flick, hot plate), electrical (foot shock), and mechanical (pinch) noxious stimuli. The time course, opioid dose-response relationship, and opioid pretreatment parameters of withdrawal hyperalgesia have been described such that it has been demonstrated to arise following single or chronic opioid exposure (74–76), can be detected up to five days following subcutaneous morphine injection (65,74,77), and increases in intensity with pretreatment opioid dose (72,77).

Subsequent work confirmed that the severity of withdrawal hyperalgesia increases with intermittent or naloxone-interrupted opioid dosing (57,78,79) and that its development can be prevented by N-methyl-D-aspartate (NMDA) receptor antagonism (57,63,80–83), suggesting that it is not unlike the hyperalgesia of neuropathic origin (84–86). Further characterization of the hyperalgesia confirms that although it is present during withdrawal, it also exists independent of the withdrawal syndrome, and can, in fact, be detected in the presence of opioid analgesia (87–89). It is likely that withdrawal from opioids provides the opportunity for underlying hyperalgesia to be revealed.

Clinically, the presence of increased sensitivity to pain during opioid withdrawal is well recognized by addiction clinicians, and reflected in the DSM-IVR diagnostic criteria for this opioid-induced disorder (90). Specifically, "muscle aches" is one of eight criteria (with nausea and vomiting, lacrimation or rhinorrhea, pupillary dilation, piloerection or sweating, diarrhea, yawning, fever, and insomnia) used for the diagnosis of the opioid withdrawal syndrome, and appears to refer to this hyperalgesic state. With respect to the signs and symptoms of opioid withdrawal, the text states:

> The first of these are subjective and consist of complaints of anxiety, restlessness, and an *"achy feeling"* that is often located in the back and legs, accompanied by a wish to obtain opioids ("craving") and drug-seeking behavior, along with irritability and *increased sensitivity to pain.* (p. 272)

Although better characterized in animals than in patients at the time the DSM criteria were written, increased sensitivity to pain was an acknowledged clinical symptom of the opioid withdrawal syndrome.

More recently, mechanical and thermal hyperalgesia have been characterized in healthy volunteers during acute withdrawal from opioids commonly used in clinical practice (morphine, hydromorphone, remifentanil). Areas of mechanical hyperalgesia induced by capsaicin and ES have been demonstrated to increase by 130% to 180% beginning within an hour of discontinuation of a 60 to 90 minute IV infusion of remifentanil (91,92). This effect was blocked by the administration of the NMDA receptor antagonist S-ketamine 30 minutes prior to remifentanil administration (91). Using a model of naloxone-precipitated withdrawal, our own work has shown significant decreases in CP pain threshold and tolerance following a single acute dose of IV hydromorphone (93).

Thus, an opioid addict is likely to appear hyperalgesic if experiencing opioid withdrawal. This becomes particularly relevant in the case of patients using heroin or short-acting prescription opioids, as the relatively rapid decrease in opioid blood levels following use allows for the emergence of intermittent withdrawal states. Yet, the hyperalgesia has been demonstrated to exist even when withdrawal is not present, thus withdrawal alone cannot explain the relative pain intolerance of this patient population.

### Exposure to Opioids

Increasingly, it is suggested that the relative pain intolerance noted in opioid maintained individuals is the result of ongoing opioid exposure, or OIH (for reviews, see Refs. 3,89,94). Convergent lines of preclinical and clinical evidence indicate that opioid administration not only provides a rapid and powerful analgesia, but concurrently sets into motion certain antianalgesic or hyperalgesic opponent processes, which (as noted earlier) can be observed during both opioid activity and withdrawal (79,91,94–98). The implications of this altered pain state have become of interest to clinicians involved in the prescription of opioid analgesics to chronic pain patients for fear that OIH may complicate or counteract opioid therapy (4,6,99,100).

The time course, opioid dose-response relationship, and opioid pretreatment parameters of OIH have been carefully characterized in preclinical models for over 30 years, such that it arises following single or chronic opioid exposure, can be detected up to five days following subcutaneous injection, and increases in intensity with pretreatment opioid dose (65,72,74,76,77). A biphasic response to opioid administration is described such that analgesia is an early response, followed by the longer lasting hyperalgesic state (81,101). More recent work has shown that it relies upon μ-opioid receptor activation, can be induced with opioids of differing intrinsic efficacy, and increases in severity with intermittent or naloxone-interrupted opioid dosing (78,79,81,102). Increasingly, OIH is recognized as a variant of central sensitization and, like the hyperalgesia of neuropathic origin (84,86), can be prevented by NMDA receptor antagonism and calcium channel blockers (63,80–83,103). Across this literature, it is of note that the degree of hyperalgesic response to opioid administration reported (∼30% of baseline) is quite reliable.

In that they appear to occur simultaneously by a similar mechanism (102,104–106), the development of hyperalgesia with opioid administration demands reconsideration of the well-known clinical phenomenon of analgesic tolerance. As eloquently suggested by Colpaert (104,107) and Celerier et al. (80,81,108), that which appears to be opioid analgesic tolerance, and therefore increased opioid need, may in fact be an organismic response to an opioid-induced hypersensitivity to pain. Subsequent work suggests that OIH and tolerance are, in fact, distinct neurophysiologic processes, yet, that OIH may play a role in the variable and incompletely understood phenomenon of analgesic tolerance in the clinical setting is an important idea. Analgesic tolerance has long been an untested rationale for withholding opioids in the treatment of chronic pain (109,110); appreciating that a component of apparent analgesic tolerance is OIH may lead to novel insights into the utility of chronic opioid therapy for this patient population.

From the above evidence, it appears that OIH is the most robust contributor to the hyperalgesia of opioid addicts. A patient dependent on opioids may be predisposed to hyperalgesia related to genetically imbued patterns of opioid response, or the tendency to suffer opioid withdrawal, but the event necessary for its development is the binding of exogenous opioids to the μ-opioid receptor. Changes in pain systems consequent to opioid exposure are critical to the development and clinical expression of hyperalgesia in patients with opioid addiction.

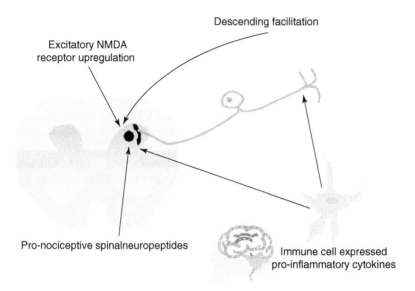

Descending facilitation

Excitatory NMDA
receptor upregulation

Pro-nociceptive spinalneuropeptides

Immune cell expressed
pro-inflammatory cytokines

**Figure 1** Theorized mechanisms of opioid-induced hyperalagesia (15). *Source*: Adapted from Ref. 3.

## What Neurobiological Substrates Underlie OIH?

Multiple neurophysiologic mechanisms for the development of OIH have been hypothesized and empirically supported (Fig. 1). Much work has been done implicating agonist activity at the excitatory ionotropic NMDA receptor on dorsal horn neurons in the development of OIH. As elegantly demonstrated in the work of Mao and colleagues (86,94,111), binding of opioids to receptors on spinal neurons induces changes such that colocalized excitatory NMDA receptors are essentially upregulated, and thus resulting in increased transmission of nociceptive signals.

Various spinal neuropeptides, distinct from excitatory amino acid systems, have also been implicated in the development of OIH. Over a decade ago, Simonnet's laboratory showed that a single dose of parenteral heroin resulted in significant release of the antiopioid neuropeptide FF from the spinal cord in rats, an effect blocked by the subsequent administration of opioid antagonist naloxone, and inducing a hyperalgesia 30% below baseline within 30 minutes (62). More recent animal work in Porreca's laboratory has demonstrated increased levels of lumbar dynorphin (a κ-opioid agonist with pronociceptive activity) following sustained spinal administration of opioid (112,113). Interestingly, the hyperalgesic effects of opioids were reversed 15 minutes following the administration of an antagonist to the neurokinin-1 receptor, the site of activity for the nociceptive neuropeptide substance P (114,115). Particularly active in pain of inflammatory origin, involvement of substance P suggests a neuroinflammatory component to the development of OIH (89).

Conversely, Porreca and colleagues have provided good preclinical evidence (98) that OIH may in fact be the result of the activation of supraspinal descending pain facilitation systems arising from μ-opioid receptor activation (102) in the rostral ventromedial medulla (RVM) (89,98,115,116). Specifically implicated are increased levels of the pronociceptive peptide cholecystokinin (CCK) in the RVM, which appear to play a role in the development of opioid analgesic tolerance as well (117). It is suggested that CCK activity in the medulla drives descending pain facilitatory mechanisms, resulting in spinal hyperalgesic responses to nociceptive input (113,118).

Neuroimmune mechanisms underlying the development of OIH have also been posited (119,120). In this model, exogenously administered opioids are theorized to bind to μ-opioid receptors located on the astrocytes of the blood-brain barrier, and result in the subsequent expression and release of proinflammatory chemokines and cytokines. In support of this hypothesis, Song and Zhao (121), and Johnston and Westbrook (122) have demonstrated that the administration of a glial cell inhibitor (fluorocitrate) reversed the hyperalgesic effect of morphine in acute and chronically treated rats up to two hours following infusion. Further, administration of the cytokine inhibitors, interleukin-1β receptor antagonist and interleukin-6 neutralizing antibody, have been shown to reverse and/or block morphine-induced hyperalgesia six days following treatment (123,124). Interestingly, coadministration of the tricyclic antidepressant amitriptyline with morphine in an animal model preserved the opioid's antinociceptive effect five days following treatment, theorized to be due to its ability to suppress opioid-induced glial cell activation and subsequent cytokine expression (125). Although the effects of spinal neuropeptides on OIH are evident acutely (15–30 minutes following treatment), immune-mediated mechanisms of OIH-reversal have been shown to be relatively enduring (5– 6 days following treatment).

As is clear from the above review, the preponderance of evidence for the existence and characteristics of OIH have been established in animal models, making it difficult to extrapolate from preclinical findings to clinical implications. Not only is pain a much more highly modulated experience in humans, but it also is not entirely clear how pain *tolerance* in humans (point of subjective intolerance of pain, an indicator of hyperalgesia) maps onto putative pain *threshold* or perception (point at which animal withdraws tail, jumps on hotplate) in animals. Further, the development of OIH has been better characterized in animals without pain or with acute pain, thus understanding of its effect and relevance in the setting of clinical addiction remain incomplete.

## Clinical Observations on OIH and Addiction

### Similarities Between Opioid-Induced Hyperalgesia and Neuropathic Pain

That hyperalgesia among methadone-maintained patients is most obvious when examined with a CP test suggests an underlying neural mechanism that may be similar or overlap the neurobiological mechanisms of chronic neuropathic pain, which in turn may have clinical implications, that is, management. The fact that OIH in these patients is most dramatically shown in the CP test suggests that there may be a common underlying mechanism between the OIH in these patients and the mechanism underlying the persistent pain in patients with neuropathic pain, i.e., central sensitization. One notable finding in the OIH among methadone-maintained patients undergoing CP tests is the changed slope, the steep rise, between pain perception and tolerance, corresponding clinically with dysesthesia in patients with, say, diabetic neuropathic pain. If central sensitization does prove to be the common underlying mechanisms for the clinical manifestations of both groups of patients, then there is a need for us to reassess our traditional understanding of these patients' clinical complaints that may, in turn, require a new attitude toward interpreting their complaints and a new approach toward treating them.

## Contribution to the Addiction Process

Still unknown and puzzling is what role hyperalgesia may have in the initiation or perpetuation of opiate addiction and what role it has in relapse after successful treatment. We know that opiate addicts are hyperalgesic and that pain is a common problem among patients on methadone maintenance, but few patients attending methadone clinics, despite their frequent pain experience, complain of hyperalgesia as such, and do not either complain of allodynia or show allodynia on examination, but why?

It is a mystery that a group of people, who are so highly physiologically dependent on opioids and are regularly exposed to high doses of opioids with daily fluctuations over a wide range of blood levels, would profess to be in need of opioids in terms of their drug hunger with little or no clinical complaints that even remotely related to hyperalgesia or allodynia on one hand, and yet show such a high degree on hyperalgesia on specific testing on the other. It is also a mystery as to why are they so hyperalgesic on one method of testing, that is, the CP test, but not on another, the ES. It is tempting to simply gloss over the observation by saying that the mechanisms underlying these tests are different but this is not a particularly satisfactory or useful explanation from the perspective of the clinician.

## Clinical Assessment of OIH in Addicts

Unfortunately, we do not yet have very adequate tools at the bedside to evaluate hyperalgesia, allodynia, and other clinically relevant manifestations of central sensitization. The few clinical hints offered by these patients are just the kind of things that clinicians have come to regard traditionally as indications of patient exaggerations and nondisease. For example, generations of clinicians have been taught that complaints and findings of pain spreading beyond the original site of injury to the contralateral side and the spread that does not follow the distribution of the peripheral nerves are indications of "nonorganic" basis and suggest that patients are exaggerating or making things up for "secondary gains" like drug seeking. Yet, these are just the type of clinical manifestations one would expect to see in central sensitization. Until we are able to more adequately detect and quantify these clinical phenomena, patients are likely to continue to suffer, especially patients with diseases both of pain and addiction. It's probably not an over statement that an addict in pain suffers thrice: once from the affliction that causes pain, once from the addiction that makes it difficult to deal with pain and once from the misunderstanding and mistreatment of their care givers. The need for a core competence in pain and in addiction for clinicians engaged in the care of these patients seems obvious.

## Suggested Clinical Guidelines for Treating OIH in Addicts

Although well-designed clinical trials are lacking, certain strategies can be recommended to help avoid or minimize the expression of OIH in the patient with addiction. First, the research literature suggests using opioid-sparing approaches to the degree possible; OIH is demonstrated to increase with opioid dose and length of exposure (126); thus, it can help to keep the maintenance opioid dose as low as is clinically effective.

Next, as is standard for opioid substitution treatment for opioid addiction, the use of long-acting opioids (i.e., methadone, buprenorphine) is indicated to minimize the expression of OIH. These agents have a more gradual onset and offset of action, avoiding the rapid escalations in opioid plasma levels that have been related to the development of OIH in clinical and preclinical settings. Additionally, investigators have shown that intermittent opioid dosing or repeated episodes of opioid withdrawal worsen OIH, thus the relatively stable plasma levels of drug afforded by long-acting opioids may help to minimize the emergence of OIH (92,127).

Another approach for opioid sparing in addicted patients is the use of adjuvant medications. The best-studied agent in this regard is the relatively weak NMDA-antagonist dextromethorphan, although, evidence for its efficacy to offset OIH in addicted patients has been mixed. Acute dextromethorphan administration has been shown to decrease the opioid-analgesic requirement (possibly due to emerging OIH) in postoperative patients (128,129) and to reduce OIH in cancer patients, but it appears less effective in consistently doing so for patients with chronic nonmalignant pain (130–133).

Recent work in our laboratory found that a five-week trial of dextromethorphan (titrated to 480 mg/day) in a well-characterized sample of MM patients was no different than placebo in improving CP threshold, CP tolerance, ES threshold, or ES tolerance, both pre and postmethadone administration (15). Notably, pain responses significantly differed by gender, with women tending to show diminished tolerance for pain with dextromethorphan therapy. The pre-clinical data of Chaplan et al. (134) show dextromethorphan to be less effective in treating formalin-induced hyperalgesia than the more potent MK801, suggesting that the weak activity of the former may account for negative findings. These conflicting data suggest that a trial of dextromethorphan may be attempted and be helpful in certain patients, but the clinician should prescribe with the understanding that it may not be effective.

Other adjuvants that have been identified as being potentially helpful in minimizing OIH in addicts and pain patients include

- propofol, due to its gabaminergic activity (135);
- COX-2 inhibitors (e.g., parecoxib, rofecoxib) for their ability to inhibit prostaglandin synthesis (136,137);
- CCK antagonists (e.g., proglumide) to block descending pain facilitatory processes (138–140);
- α2-Receptor agonists (e.g., clonidine), which appeared to attenuate OIH in a small sample of healthy human subjects (105).

Of increasing interest in the literature is the use of low-dose opioid antagonists in conjunction with opioid agonists to counteract the development of OIH (141–145). In two recent randomized clinical trials of pain patients with osteoarthritis (146) and low back pain (147), investigators reported significant benefits for pain relief over time and diminished physical withdrawal with the combination of oxycodone-plus-low-dose naltrexone (2–4 µg/day) versus oxycodone alone. It is theorized that the efficacy of low-dose opioid antagonists in preventing OIH is related to the suppression of G-protein switching in the presence of opioid agonist (148).

## Some Remaining Unresolved Issues and Future Questions

Many questions remain about the development and treatment of OIH in addicted patients prescribed ongoing opioid therapy. In that many chronic pain syndromes include a significant neuropathic component, it is conceivable that any hyperalgesia induced by opioid therapy might contribute to this neuropathy, thereby worsening the experience of pain.

The time-course of OIH development also is unclear. Opioid withdrawal-related hyperalgesia can be elicited within hours of opioid exposure (91,93,96) and OIH appears to develop after relatively short courses of intraoperative opioid administration (149–151). As previously noted, limited evidence from our laboratory indicates that the development of OIH may vary among different opioid medications, especially those that differ in intrinsic activity (e.g., methadone vs. buprenorphine) (11). Therefore, which treatment opioids are more or less likely to induce OIH, and at what point following opioid exposure, are important but still unanswered questions.

Finally, the presentation of hyperalgesia in street addicts or prescription opioid abusers remains undescribed. As noted, methadone maintenance imparts a relative degree of physiological and social stability to patients not enjoyed by untreated opioid addicts. Based upon the tendency to use short-acting high-potency opioids and to experience opioid withdrawal, it might be expected that the hyperalgesia of untreated opioid addicts is even more robust than that of those on methadone therapy.

## CONCLUSIONS

Decades of use have shown that maintenance opioids are highly effective for the treatment of opioid addiction. OIH does not appear to complicate the management of addiction at the clinical level, although its role in perpetuating opioid use remains unknown. Regardless, fears of inducing OIH should not limit the pre-scribing of treatment opioids when clinically necessary. Yet, the development of OIH has been consistently demonstrated following opioid administration in animal models, and increasingly in humans with and without pain. Theorized factors underlying the individual development of OIH range from genetic-influences to behavioral opioid responses, but exposure to opioids appears requisite.

What is clearly evident from the literature is that opioid addicts do have decreased tolerance for pain, a component of which can likely be attributed to OIH. Its expression becomes most problematic clinically when the patient has a painful condition that requires analgesic treatment. Complaints of pain from opioid addicts are typically met with a certain degree of skepticism, and often interpreted more as drug-seeking than legitimate. OIH provides an explanation not only for why their pain persists despite notable opioid blood levels of opioids, but also for the often diffuse and atypical presentation of the pain itself. Interventions aimed at limiting or minimizing the development of OIH in this population remain essentially untested, although the use of long-acting opioids and opioid-sparing strategies appear to be rational approaches suggested by the preclinical data. Definitive management strategies will have to await a better understanding of what role OIH really plays in addiction to opioids.

## REFERENCES

1. Mitchell SW. Characteristics. New York: The Century Company, 1905:21.
2. Albutt C. On the abuse of hypodermic injections of morphia. Practitioner 1870; 3:327–330.
3. Angst MJ, Clark JD. Opioid-induced hyperalgesia: a qualitative systematic review. Anesthesiology 2006; 104:6570–687.
4. Chang G, Chen L, Mao J. Opioid tolerance and hyperalgesia. Med Clin North Am 2007; 91:199–211.
5. Chu LF, Angst MS, Clark JD. Opioid-induced hyperalgesia in humans: molecular mechanisms and clinical considerations. Clin J Pain 2008; 24:479–496.
6. Koppert W, Schmelz M. The impact of opioid-induced hyperalgesia for post-operative pain. Best Pract Res Clin Anesthesiol 2007; 21:65–83.
7. Martin J, Inglis J. Pain tolerance and narcotic addiction. Br J Sociol Clin Psychol 1965; 4:224–229.

8. Ho A, Dole V. Pain perception in drug-free and in methadone-maintained human ex-addicts. Proc Soc Exp Biol Med 1979; 162:392–395.
9. Compton MA. Cold pressor pain tolerance in opiate and cocaine abusers: Correlates of drug type and use status. J Pain Symptom Manage 1994; 9:462–473.
10. Compton P, Charuvastra C, Kintaudi K, et al. Pain responses in methadone-maintained opioid abusers. J Pain Symptom Manag 2000; 20:237–245.
11. Compton P, Charuvastra VC, Ling W. Pain intolerance in opioid-maintained former opiate addicts: effect of long-acting maintenance agent. Drug Alcohol Depend 2001; 63:139–146.
12. Doverty M, White JM, Somogyi AA, et al. Hyperalgesic responses in methadone maintenance patients. Pain 2001; 90:91–96.
13. Doverty M, Somogyi AA, White JM, et al. Methadone maintenance patients are cross-tolerant to the antinociceptive effects of morphine. Pain 2001; 93:155–163.
14. Schall U, Katta T, Pries E, et al. Pain perception of intravenous heroin users on maintenance therapy with levomethadone. Pharmacopsychiatry 1996; 29:176–179.
15. Compton PA, Ling W, Torrington MA. Lack of effect of chronic dextromethorphan on experimental pain tolerance in methadone-maintained patients. Addict Biol 2008; 13:393–402.
16. Athanasos P, Smith CS, White JM, et al.. Methadone maintenance patients are cross tolerant to the antinociceptive effects of very high plasma morphine concentrations. Pain 2006; 120:267–275.
17. Pud D, Cohen D, Lawental E, et al. Opioids and abnormal pain perception: new evidence from a study of chronic opioid addicts and healthy subjects. Drug Alcohol Depend 2006; 82:218–223.
18. Mogil JS, Kest B, Sadowski B, et al. Differential genetic mediation of sensitivity to morphine in genetic models of opiate antinociception: influence of nociceptive assay. J Pharmacol Exp Ther 1996; 276:532–544.
19. Mogil JS, Wilson SG, Bon K, et al. Heritability of nociception I: responses of 11 inbred mouse strains on 12 measures of nociception. Pain 1999; 80:67–82.
20. Elmer GI. Differences in morphine reinforcement property in two inbred rat strains: associations with cortical receptors, behavioral activity, analgesia and the cataleptic effects of morphine. Psychopharmacology (Berlin) 1993; 112:183–188.
21. Elmer GI, Pieper JO, Goldberg SR, et al. Opioid operant self-administration, analgesia, stimulation and respiratory depression in mu-deficient mice. Psychopharmacology (Berlin) 1995; 117:23–31.
22. Elmer GI, Pieper JO, Negus SS, et al. Genetic variance in nociception and its relationship to the potency of morphine-induced analgesia in thermal and chemical tests. Pain 1998; 75:129–240.
23. Oliverio A, Castellano C, Eleftheriou BE. Morphine sensitivity and tolerance: a genetic investigation in the mouse. Psychopharmacologia 1975; 42:219–224.
24. Semenova S, Kuzmin A, Zvartau E. Strain differences in the analgesic and reinforcing action of morphine in mice. Pharmacol Biochem Behav 1995; 50:17–21.
25. Oliverio A, Castellano C. Genotype-dependent sensitivity and tolerance to morphine and heroin: dissociation between opiate-induced running and analgesia in the mouse. Psychopharmacologia 1974; 39:13–22.
26. Wilson SG, Smith SB, Chesler EJ, et al. The heritability of antinociception: common pharmacogenetic mediation of five neurochemically distinct analgesics. J Pharmacol Exp Ther 2003; 304:547–559.

27. Lariviere WR, Wilson SG, Laughlin TM, et al. Heritability of nociception. III. Genetic relationships among commonly used assays of nociception and hypersensitivity. Pain 2002; 97:75–86.

28. Liang DY, Guo T, Liao G, et al. Chronic pain and genetic background interact and influence opioid analgesia, tolerance, and physical dependence. Pain 2006; 121: 232–240.

29. Brase DA, Loh HH, Way EL. Comparison of the effects of morphine on locomotor activity, analgesia and primary and protracted physical dependence in six mouse strains. J Pharmacol Exp Ther 1977; 201:368–374.

30. Racagni G, Bruno F, Iuliano E, et al. Differential sensitivity to morphine-induced analgesia and motor activity in two inbred strains of mice: behavioral and biochemical correlations. J Pharmacol Exp Ther 1979; 209:111–116.

31. Gwynn GJ, Domino EF. Genotype-dependent behavioral sensitivity to mu vs. kappa opiate agonists. II. Antinociceptive tolerance and physical dependence. J Pharmacol Exp Ther 1984; 231:312–316.

32. Moskowitz AS, Terman GW, Carter KR, et al. Analgesic, locomotor and lethal effects of morphine in the mouse: strain comparisons. Brain Res 1985; 361:46–51.

33. Belknap JK, Mogil JS, Helms ML, et al. Localization to chromosome 10 of a locus influencing morphine analgesia in crosses derived from C57BL/6 and DBA/2 strains. Life Sci 1995; 57:PL117–PL124.

34. Berrettini WH, Ferraro TN, Alexander RC, et al. Quantitative trait loci mapping of three loci controlling morphine preference using inbred mouse strains. Nat Genet 1994; 7:54–58.

35. Liang DY, Liao G, Lighthall GK, et al. Genetic variants of the P-glycoprotein gene Abcb1b modulate opioid-induced hyperalgesia, tolerance and dependence. Pharmacogenet Genomics 2006; 16:825–835.

36. Petruzzi R, Ferraro TN, Kürschner VC, et al. The effects of repeated morphine exposure on mu opioid receptor number and affinity in C57BL/6J and DBA/2J mice. Life Sci 1997; 61:2057–2064.

37. Mogil JS, Przemyslaw M, Flodman P, et al. One or two genetic loci mediate high opiate analgesia in selectively bred mice. Pain 1995; 60:125–135.

38. Moskowitz AS, Goodman RR. Autoradiographic analysis of mu1, mu2, and delta opioid binding in the central nervous system of C57BL/6BY and CXBK (opioid receptor-deficient) mice. Brain Res 1985; 360:108–116.

39. Compton P, Alarcon M, Geschwin D. Role of the m-opioid receptor gene in human pain tolerance and opioid addiction. Drug Alcohol Depend 2001; 63:S30—S31.

40. Edwards RR. Genetic predictors of acute and chronic pain. Curr Rheumatol Rep 2006; 8:411–417.

41. Mogil JS, Yu L, Basbaum AI. Pain genes? Natural variation and transgenic mutants. Annu Rev Neurosci 2000; 23:777–811.

42. Oertel B, Lötsch J. Genetic mutations that prevent pain: implications for future pain medication. Pharmacogenomics 2008; 9:179–194.

43. Stamer UM, Stüber F. Genetic factors in pain and its treatment. Curr Opin Anaesthesiol 2007; 20:478–484.

44. Flores CM, Mogil JS. The pharmacogenetics of analgesia: toward a genetically-based approach to pain management. Pharmacogenomics 2001; 2:177–194.

45. Lötsch J, Skarke C, Liefhold J, et al. Genetic predictors of the clinical response to opioid analgesics: clinical utility and future perspectives. Clin Pharmacokinet 2004; 43:983–1013.

46. Stamer UM, Stüber F. The pharmacogenetics of analgesia. Expert Opin Pharmacother 2007; 8:2235–2245.

47. Mayer P, Höllt V. Pharmacogenetics of opioid receptors and addiction. Pharmacogenet Genomics 2006; 16:1–7.

48. Ikeda K, Ide S, Han W, et al. How individual sensitivity to opiates can be predicted by genetic analyses. Trends Pharmacol Sci 2005; 26:311–317.

49. Kest B, Hopkins E, Palmese CA, et al. Genetic variation in morphine analgesic tolerance: a survey of 11 inbred mouse strains. Pharmacol Biochem Behav 2002; 73:821–828.

50. Kest B, Palmese CA, Hopkins E, et al. Naloxone-precipitated withdrawal jumping in 11 inbred mouse strains: evidence for common genetic mechanisms in acute and chronic morphine physical dependence. Neuroscience 2002; 115:463–469.

51. Kest B, Palmese CA, Juni A, et al. Mapping of a quantitative trait locus for morphine withdrawal severity. Mamm Genome 2004; 15:610–617.

52. Lötsch J, Geisslinger G. Relevance of frequent mu-opioid receptor polymorphisms for opioid activity in healthy volunteers. Pharmacogenomics J 2006; 6:200–210.

53. Kim H, Neubert JK, Miguel AS, et al. Genetic influence on variability in human acute experimental pain sensitivity associated with gender, ethnicity and psychological temperament. Pain 2004; 109:488–496.

54. Caterina MJ, Leffler A, Malmberg AB, et al. Impaired nociception and pain sensation in mice lacking the capsaicin receptor. Science 2000; 14:306–313.

55. McKemy DD, Neuhausser WM, Julius D. Identification of a cold receptor reveals a general role for TRP channels in thermosensation. Nature 2002; 7:52–58.

56. Mogil JS, Ritchie J, Smith SB, et al. Melanocortin-1 receptor gene variants affect pain and mu-opioid analgesia in mice and humans. J Med Genet 2005; 42:583–587.

57. Li X, Angst MS, Clark D. A murine model of opioid-induced hyperalgesia. Brain Res Mol Brain Res 2001; 86:56–62.

58. Liebmann P, Lehofer M, Schonauer-Cejpek M, et al. Pain sensitivity in former opioid addicts. Lancet 1994; 344:1031–1032.

59. Liebmann P, Lehofer M, Moser M, et al. Persistent analgesia in former opiate addicts is resistant to blockade of endogenous opioids. Biol Psychiatry 1997; 42:962–964.

60. Liebmann P, Lehofer M, Moser M, et al. Nervousness and pain sensitivity. II. Changed relation in ex-addicts as a predictor for early relapse. Psychiatry Res 1998; 79:55–58.

61. Prosser JM, Steinfeld M, Cohen LJ, et al. Abnormal heat and pain perception in remitted heroin dependence months after detoxification from methadone-maintenance. Drug Alcohol Depend 2008; 95:237–244.

62. Devillers JP, Boisserie F, Laulin JP, et al. Simultaneous activation of spinal anti-opioid system (neuropeptide FF) and pain facilitatory circuitry by stimulation of opioid receptors in rats. Brain Res 1995; 700:173–181.

63. Dunbar SA, Pulai IJ. Repetitive opioid abstinence causes progressive hyperalgesia sensitive to $N$-methyl-D-aspartate receptor blockade in the rat. J Pharmacol Exp Ther 1998; 284:678–686.

64. Ekblom M, Hammerlund-Udenaes M, Paalzow L. Modeling of tolerance development and rebound effect during different intravenous administrations of morphine to rats. J Pharmacol Exp Ther 1993; 266:244–252.

65. Grilly DM, Gowans GC. Acute morphine dependence: effects observed in shock and light discrimination tasks. Psychopharmacology (Berlin) 1986; 88:500–504.

66. Johnson SM, Duggan AW. Tolerance and dependence of dorsal horn neurons of the cat: the role of the opiate receptors of the substantia gelatinosa. Neuropharmacology 1981; 20:1033–1038.

67. Laulin JP, Larcher A, Celerier E, et al. Long-lasting increased pain sensitivity in rat following exposure to heroin for the first time. Eur J Neurosci 1998; 10:782–785.

68. Donnerer J. Primary sensory neurons and naloxone-precipitated morphine withdrawal. Br J Pharmacol 1989; 86:767–772.

69. Kaplan H, Fields HL. Hyperalgesia during acute opioid abstinence: evidence for a nociceptive facilitating function of the rostral ventromedial medulla. J Neurosci 1991; 11:1433–1439.

70. Martin WR, Eades CG. A comparison between acute and chronic physical dependence in the chronic spinal dog. J Pharmacol Exp Ther 1964; 146:385–394.

71. Martin WR, Gilbert PE, Jasinski PE, et al. An analysis of naltrexone precipitated abstinence in morphine-dependent chronic spinal dogs. J Pharmacol Exp Ther 1987; 240:565–570.

72. Tilson HA, Rech RH, Stolman S. Hyperalgesia during withdrawal as a means of measuring the degree of dependence in morphine dependent rats. Psychopharmacologia 1973; 28:287–300.

73. Yaksh TL, Harty GJ, Onofrio BM. High doses of spinal morphine produce a nonopiate receptor-mediated hyperesthesia: clinical and theoretic implications. Anesthesiology 1986; 64:590–597.

74. Bederson JB, Fields HL, Barbaro NM. Hyperalgesia during naloxone-precipitated withdrawal from morphine is associated with increased on-cell activity in the rostral ventromedial medulla. Somatosens Mot Res 1990; 7:185–203.

75. Goldfarb J, Kaplan EI, Jenkins HR. Interaction of morphine and naloxone in acute spinal cats. Neuropharmacology 1978; 17:569–575.

76. Kim DH, Barbaro NM, Fields HL. Dose response relationship for hyperalgesia following naloxone precipitated withdrawal from morphine. Soc Neurosci Abstr 1988; 14:174.

77. Kim DH, Fields HL, Barbaro NM. Morphine analgesia and acute physical dependence: rapid onset of two opposing, dose-related processes. Brain Res 1990; 516:37–40.

78. Ibuki T, Dunbar SA, Yaksh TL. Effect of transient naloxone antagonism in tolerance development in rats receiving continuous spinal morphine infusion. Pain 1997; 70:125–132.

79. Li X, Angst MS, Clark D. Opioid-induced hyperalgesia incisional pain. Anaesth Analg 2001; 93:204–209.

80. Celerier E, Laulin JP, Larcher A, et al. Evidence for opiate-activated NMDA processes masking opiate analgesia in rats. Brain Res 1999; 847:18–25.

81. Celerier E, Rivat C, Jun Y, et al. Long-lasting hyperalgesia induced by fentanyl in rats: preventative effect of ketamine. Anesthesiology 2000; 92:465–472.

82. Dunbar S, Yaksh TL. Concurrent spinal infusion of MK801 blocks spinal tolerance and dependence induced by chronic intrathecal morphine in the rat. Anesthesiology 1996; 84:1177–1188.

83. Larcher A, Laulin JP, Celerier E, et al. Acute tolerance associated with a single opiate administration: involvement of N-methyl-D-aspertate-dependent pain facilitatory systems. Neuroscience 1998; 84:583–589.

84. Mao J, Price DD, Mayer DJ. Experimental mononeuropathy reduces the anti-nociceptive effects of morphine: implications for common intracellular mechanisms involved in morphine tolerance and neuropathic pain. Pain 1995; 1:353–364.
85. Mao J, Price DD, Mayer DJ. Mechanisms of hyperalgesia and morphine tolerance: a current view of their possible interactions. Pain 1995; 62:259–274.
86. Mayer DJ, Mao J, Holt J, et al. Cellular mechanisms of neuropathic pain, morphine tolerance, and their interactions. Proc Natl Acad Sci USA 1999; 96:7731–7736.
87. Chu L, Angst M, Clark, D. Opioids in non-cancer pain: measurement of opioid-induced tolerance and hyperalgesia in pain patients on chronic opioid therapy. J Pain 2004; 5:S73.
88. Holtman JR, Wala EP. Characterization of morphine-induced hyperalgesia in male and female rats. Pain 2005;114:62–70.
89. Ossipov MH, Lai J, King T, et al. Underlying mechanisms of pronociceptive consequences of prolonged morphine exposure. Pept Sci 2005; 80:319–324.
90. American Psychiatric Association. Diagnostic and Statistical Manual of Mental Disorders (DSM-IV-TR)4th ed., Text Revision. Arlington, VA: American Psychiatric Association, 2000.
91. Angst MS, Koppert W, Pahl I, et al. Short-term infusion of the mu-opioid agonist remifentanil in humans causes hyperalgesia during withdrawal. Pain. 2003; 106: 49–57.
92. Hood DD, Curry R, Eisenach JC. Intravenous remifentanil produces withdrawal hyperalgesia in volunteers with capsaicin-induced hyperalgesia. Anesth Analg 2003; 97:810–815.
93. Compton P, Athanasos P, Elashoff D. Withdrawal hyperalgesia after acute opioid physical dependence in nonaddicted humans: a preliminary study. J Pain 2003; 4:511–519.
94. Mao J. Opioid-induced abnormal pain sensitivity: implications in clinical opioid therapy. Pain 2002; 100:213–217.
95. Chu LF, Clark DJ, Angst MS. Opioid tolerance and hyperalgesia in chronic pain patients after one month of oral morphine therapy: a preliminary prospective study. J Pain 2006; 7:43–48.
96. Koppert W, Angst M, Alsheimer M, et al. Naloxone provokes similar pain facilitation as observed after short-term infusion of remifentanil in humans. Pain 2003; 106:91–99.
97. Simonnet G. Opioids: from analgesia to anti-hyperalgesia? Pain 2005; 118:8–9.
98. Vanderah TW, Ossipov MH, Lai J, et al.. Mechanisms of opioid–induced pain and antinociceptive tolerance: descending facilitation and spinal dynorphin. Pain 2001; 92:5–9.
99. Mercadante S, Ferrera P, Villari P, et al. Hyperalgesia: an emerging iatrogenic syndrome. J Pain Symptom Manage 2003; 26:769–775.
100. Wilder-Smith OH, Arendt-Nielsen L. Postoperative hyperalgesia: its clinical importance and relevance. Anesthesiology 2006; 104:601–607.
101. Van Elstraete AC, Sitbon P, Trabold F, et al. A single dose of intrathecal morphine in rats induces long-lasting hyperalgesia: The protective effect of prior administration of ketamine. Anesth analg 2005; 101:1750–1756.
102. Gardell LR, King T, Ossipov MH, et al. Opioid receptor-mediated hyperalgesia and antinociceptive tolerance induced by sustained opiate delivery. Neurosci Lett 2006; 396:4449.

103. Richebe P, Rivat C, Creton C, et al. Nitrous oxide revisited. Anesthesiology 2005; 105:845–854.
104. Colpaert FC. System theory of pain and of opiate analgesia: no tolerance to opiates. Pharmacol Rev 1996; 48:355–402.
105. Laulin JP, Celerier E, Larcher A, et al. Opiate tolerance to daily heroin administration: An apparent phenomenon associated with enhanced pain sensitivity. Neuroscience 1999; 89:631–636.
106. Mao J. Opioid-induced abnormal pain sensitivity. Curr Pain Headache Rep 2006; 10: 67–70.
107. Colpaert FC. Mechanisms of opioid-induced pain and antinociceptive tolerance: signal transduction. Pain 2002; 95:287–288.
108. Celerier E, Laulin JP, Corcuff JB, et al. Progressive enhancement of delayed hyperalgesia induced by repeated heroin administration: a sensitization process. J Neurosci 2001; 21:4074–4080.
109. Finnerup NB, Otto M, McQuay HJ, et al. Algorithm for neuropathic pain treatment: an evidence based proposal. Pain 2005; 118:289–305.
110. Foley KM. Opioids and chronic neuropathic pain. N Engl J Med 2003; 348: 1279–1281.
111. Mao J, Price DD, Mayer DJ. Thermal hyperalgesia in association with the development of morphine tolerance in rats: roles of excitatory amino acids receptors and protein kinase C. J Neurosci 1994; 14:2301–2312.
112. Gardell LR, Wang R, Burgess SE, et al. Sustained morphine exposure induces a spinal dynorphin-dependent enhancement of excitatory transmitter release from primary afferent fibers. J Neurosci 2002; 22:6747–6755.
113. Vanderah TW, Gardell LR, Burgess SE, et al. Dynorphin promotes abnormal pain and spinal opioid antinociceptive tolerance. J Neurosci 2000; 20:7074–7079.
114. King T, Gardell LR, Wang R, et al. Role of NK-1 neurotransmission in opioid-induced hyperalgesia. Pain 2005; 116:276–288.
115. King T, Ossipov MH, Vanderah TW, et al. Is paradoxical pain induced by sustained opioid exposure an underlying mechanism of opioid antinociceptive tolerance? Neurosignals 2005; 14:194–205.
116. Ossipov MH, Lai J, King T, et al. Antinociceptive and nociceptive actions of opioids. J Neurobiol 2004; 61:146–148.
117. Xie JY, Herman DS, Stiller CO, et al. Cholecystokinin in the rostral ventromedial medulla mediates opioid-induced hyperalgesia and antinociceptive tolerance. J Neurosci 2005; 25:409–416.
118. Vanderah T, Suenaga N, Ossipov M, et al. Tonic descending facilitation from the rostral ventromedial medulla mediates opioid-induced abnormal pain and antinociceptive tolerance. J Neurosci 2001; 21:279–286.
119. De Leo JA, Tanga FY, Tawfik VL. Neuroimmune activation and neuro-inflammation in chronic pain and opioid tolerance/hyperalgesia. Neuroscientist 2004; 10:40–52.
120. Watkins LR, Maier SF. The pain of being sick: Implications of immune-to-brain communication for understanding pain. Annu Rev Psychol 2000; 51:29–57.
121. Song P, Zhao ZQ. The involvement of glial cells in the development of morphine tolerance. Neurosci Res 2001; 39:281–286.
122. Johnston IN, Westbrook RF. Inhibition of morphine analgesia by LPS: role of opioid and NMDA receptors and spinal glia. Behav Brain Res 2005; 156:75–83.

123. Johnston IN, Milligan ED, Wieseler-Frank J. A role for proinflammatory cytokines and fractalkine in analgesia, tolerance, and subsequent pain facilitation induced by chronic intrathecal morphine. J Neurosci 2004; 24:7353–7365.
124. Raghavendra V, Rutkowski MD, DeLeo JA. The role of spinal neuroimmune activation in morphine tolerance/hyperalgesia in neuropathic and sham-operated rats. J Neurosci 2002; 22:9980–9989.
125. Tai YH, Wang YH, Wang JJ, et al. Amitriptyline suppresses neuroinflammation and up-regulates glutamate transporters in morphine-tolerant rats. Pain 2006; 124:77–86.
126. Cohen SP, Christo PJ, Wang S, et al. The effect of opioid dose and treatment duration on the perception of a painful standardized clinical stimulus. Reg Anesth Pain Med 2008; 33:199–206.
127. Sweitzer SR, Allen CP, Zissen MH, et al. Mechanical allodynia and thermal hyperalgesia upon acute opioid withdrawal in the neonatal rat. Pain 2004; 110:269–280.
128. Helmy SA, Bali A. The effect of the preemptive use of the NMDA receptor antagonist dextromethorphan on postoperative analgesic requirements. Anesth Analg 2001; 92:739–744.
129. Weinbroum A, Rudick V, Paret G, et al. The role of dextromethorphan in pain control. Can J Anaesthia 2000; 47:585–596.
130. Dudgeon DJ, Bruera E, Gagnon B, et al. A phase III randomized, double-blind, placebo-controlled study evaluating dextromethorphan plus slow-release morphine for chronic cancer pain relief in terminally ill patients. J Pain Symptom Manage 2007; 33:365–371.
131. Galer BS, Lee D, Ma T, et al. MorphiDex (morphine sulfate/dextromethorphan hydrobromide combination) in the treatment of chronic pain: three multicenter, randomized, double-blind, controlled clinical trials fail to demonstrate enhanced opioid analgesia or reduction in tolerance. Pain 2005; 115:284–295.
132. Haugan F, Rygh LJ, Tjølsen A. Ketamine blocks enhancement of spinal long-term potentiation in chronic opioid treated rats. Acta Anaesthesiol Scand 2008; 52: 681–687.
133. Heiskanen T, Härtel B, Dahl ML, et al. Analgesic effects of dextromethorphan and morphine in patients with chronic pain. Pain 2002; 96:261–267.
134. Chaplan SR, Malmberg AB, Yaksh TL. Efficacy of spinal NMDA receptor antagonism in formalin hyperalgesia and nerve injury evoked allodynia in the rat. J Pharmacol Exp Ther 1997; 280:829–838.
135. Singler B, Tröster A, Manering N, et al. Modulation of remifentanil-induced postinfusion hyperalgesia by propofol. Anesth Analg 2007; 104:1397–1403.
136. Joshi W, Connelly NR, Reuben SS, et al. An evaluation of the safety and efficacy of administering rofecoxib for postoperative pain management. Anesth Analg 2003; 97:35–38.
137. Tröster A, Sittl R, Singler B, et al. Modulation of remifentanil-induced analgesia and postinfusion hyperalgesia by parecoxib in humans. Anesthesiology 2006; 105:1016–1023.
138. Bernstein ZP, Yucht S, Battista E, et al. Proglumide as a morphine adjunct in cancer pain management. J Pain Symptom Manage 1998; 15:314–320.
139. McCleane GJ. The cholecystokinin antagonist proglumide enhances the analgesic effect of dihydrocodeine. Clin J Pain 2003; 19:200–201.
140. McCleane GJ. Cholecystokinin antagonists a new way to improve the analgesia from old analgesics? Curr Pharm Des 2004; 10:303–314.

141. Carroll IR, Angst MS, Clark JD. Management of perioperative pain in patients chronically consuming opioids. Reg Anesth Pain Med 2004; 29:576–591.
142. Cepeda MS, Alvarez H, Morales O, et al. Addition of ultralow dose naloxone to postoperative morphine PCA: unchanged analgesia and opioid requirement but decreased incidence of opioid side effects. Pain 2004; 107:41–46.
143. Terner JM, Barrett AC, Lomas LM, et al. Influence of low doses of naltrexone on morphine antinociception and morphine tolerance in male and female rats of four strains. Pain 2006; 122:90–101.
144. Wang HY, Friedman E, Olmstead MC, et al. Ultra-low-dose naloxone suppresses opioid tolerance, dependence and associated changes in mu opioid receptor-G protein coupling and Gbetagamma signaling. Neuroscience 2005; 135:247–261.
145. Webster LR. Oxytrex: an oxycodone and ultra-low-dose naltrexone formulation. Expert Opin Investig Drugs 2007; 16:1277–1283.
146. Chindalore VL, Craven RA, Yu KP, et al. Adding ultralow-dose naltrexone to oxycodone enhances and prolongs analgesia: a randomized, controlled trial of Oxytrex. J Pain 2005; 6:392–399.
147. Webster LR, Butera PG, Moran LV, et al. Oxytrex minimizes physical dependence while providing effective analgesia: a randomized controlled trial in low back pain. J Pain 2006; 7:937–946.
148. Sloan P, Harmann S. Ultra-low-dose opioid antagonists to enhance opioid analgesia. J Opioid Manage 2006; 2:295–304.
149. Chia YY, Liu K, Wang JJ, et al. Intraoperative high dose fentanyl induces post-operative fentanyl tolerance. Can J Anaesth 1999; 46:872–827.
150. Cooper DW, Lindsay SL, Ryall DM, et al. Does intrathecal fentanyl produce acute cross-tolerance to IV morphine? Br J Anaesth 1997; 78:311–313.
151. Guignard B, Bossard AE, Coste C, et al. Acute opioid tolerance: intraoperative remifentanil increases postoperative pain and morphine requirement. Anesthesiology 2000; 93:409–417.

# 7

# Practical Management of Opioid-Induced Hyperalgesia in the Primary Care Setting

**Bill McCarberg**

*Kaiser Permanente, Chronic Pain Management Program,
University of California, San Diego, California, U.S.A.*

## INTRODUCTION

The management of persistent pain in primary care is complicated and time consuming. Despite a growing knowledge about the pathophysiology of pain, management remains an elusive goal. When surveyed, only 34% of internists reported that they felt comfortable with their abilities to manage patients with persistent pain (1). Increasingly, opioids have been used to treat persistent noncancer pain. Recent IMS data shows that hydrocodone products are the most widely prescribed drugs in the United States, largely from primary care (2). In a recent article, Ballantyne and Mao wrote that the most difficult issue now facing by physicians is "...whether and how to prescribe opioid therapy for chronic pain that is not associated with terminal disease, including pain experienced by the increasing number of patients with cancer in remission (3)."

The well-established efficacy of opioids has been challenged by a variety of clinical issues including lack of long-term efficacy, side effects, addiction, and the development of tolerance among others. Relatively new on this list of problems is opioid-induced hyperalgesia (OIH). Why hyperalgesia is important to the primary care provider and what to do about it will be explored in this

**Table 1**  Chronic Conditions Treated by Primary Care Physicians Versus Other Specialists

| Conditions | Treated by primary care physicians (%) | Treated by other specialists (%) |
| --- | --- | --- |
| Arteriosclerotic cardiovascular disease (ASCVD) | 86 | 14 |
| Stroke | 91 | 9 |
| Hypertension | 92 | 8 |
| Diabetes mellitus | 90 | 10 |
| Chronic obstructive pulmonary disease (COPD) | 89 | 11 |
| Asthma | 94 | 6 |

chapter. The other chapters of this book go into much greater detail, yet this chapter will be a primary care guide to the topic.

## CHRONIC ILLNESS IN PRIMARY CARE

All primary care physicians must treat patients with a variety of chronic diseases. In fact most chronic illness is principally managed at the primary care level (Table 1) (4).

Even complicated conditions such as diabetes, which requires multiple drugs, behavior management, home glucose monitoring, and patient decision making with sliding insulin scales, can easily be handled in a primary care setting. OIH is a complicated topic with difficult diagnostic issues and uncertain pathophysiology making primary care uneasy about caring for these patients. The number of patients with persistent pain problems taking opioids makes it critical that primary care providers become familiar with this topic. Specialty referral for evaluation and treatment may be necessary for some patients, but the hallmark of successful management of OIH will be the education of the primary care provider.

## CLINICAL PRACTICE

There are many stresses that influence practice in primary care. Time is the most valuable commodity. Dealing with multiple problems at a simple visit is now a standard practice. Primary care providers are intelligent and efficient but do not have the fund of knowledge, the background, or experience to deal with many complicated medical problems. Primary care providers have become good at diabetes management through education, simple algorithms, and outcomes that are easy to measure and interpret.

It is vital that primary care clinicians learn about OIH and manage the patients with hyperalgesia, but this will only be accomplished with a straightforward, easy to understand approach. Pathophysiology, even if not fully understood, must be simplified with examples representing application in a clinical practice. Uncertainty with difficult decisions and frequent follow-up appointments are the norm in primary care, yet it must be clear what each appointment is attempting to accomplish and how to measure success. The following discussion will concentrate on making OIH understandable to a practitioner with little background in pain and just the basic knowledge of opioid analgesia mechanisms.

The main questions that arise concerning OIH in the primary care setting are:

1. Making the diagnosis—When should I be thinking about OIH?
2. Pathophysiology—Why does it occur?
3. Consequences of ignoring the problem—Why is it important to me?
4. Management—What do I do about it?
5. Recognizing limitations and need for referral—When do I need help?

If the above questions can be answered simply and reasonably, then OIH can be managed in the primary care setting. With recent surveys suggesting 75 to 105 million Americans experience pain daily or intermittently (5–7), and with the prevalence of opioid use among primary care providers, this is a topic of great concern. Given the number of patients with persistent pain requires that primary care assume management, since there are not enough specialists to deal with the potential referral base.

## Making the Diagnosis—When Should I Be Thinking About Hyperalgesia

The essential defining characteristic of hyperalgesia is increased pain for a given stimulus. Prolonged administration of opioids can result in a paradoxical increase in atypical pain that appears to be unrelated to the original nociceptive stimulus. Clinicians should suspect OIH when the opioid treatment effect lessens in the absence of disease progression, particularly if found in the context of unexplained pain reports or diffuse allodynia unassociated with the site of injury.

This may present as a patient on chronic opioid therapy for a persistent pain problem and developing a new injury or pain. The amount of pain described appears to be out of proportion to the trauma or injury. Another clinical presentation may be the patient's persistent pain worsening. Despite escalating doses of opioids, the pain does not improve and the pain has characteristics different from those of the original pain syndrome, for example, pain arising in different locations, becoming more diffuse in nature, and often spreading beyond the original disease location.

Recognition of the phenomenon of OIH in the clinical setting is a challenge and requires considering a differential diagnosis, which includes the following five conditions that could mimic hyperalgesia. Each of these conditions would have a different treatment path.

1.  Increase in the original pain-producing pathology—if the patient has cancer, has there been progression of the disease including metastasis? If the patient has degenerative disc disease, has there been further progression of the underlying degeneration? In a patient with osteoporosis and known compression fractures, has there been a new compression fracture even without trauma? The treatment would be to find the pathology and treat the generator of the pain. In this case, the opioid should be increased during the workup.
2.  Flare of original pain pathology—pain, even persistent pain waxes and wanes. Is the increased pain just a predictable flare? Has the patient done more activity or has there been a change in the weather or sleep, which has impacted pain? The treatment would consist of advise on pain flare management with activity pacing, scaling back exercise during weather changes, or practicing good sleep hygiene. Opioid doses should not change despite increasing pain scores.
3.  Opioid tolerance—state of adaptation in which exposure to a drug induces changes that result in a decrease of the drug's effects over time. Complex intracellular neural mechanisms including opioid receptor desensitization and downregulation are believed to be major mechanisms underlying opioid tolerance. The best treatment would be to increase the opioid to adjust for tolerance.
4.  Substance abuse—complex phenomenon involving psychological, genetic, environmental, and behavioral factors. Addiction is characterized by craving, compulsive use, and continued use of the opioid despite harm. Addiction is difficult to recognize in some patients, but it is common to see escalating doses of opioids with deterioration in function. When suspecting opioid addiction, withdrawal from the medication and treatment by substance abuse specialist is warranted. This issue is further discussed in other chapters in this book.
5.  Increased pain caused by a non-pain condition—escalating opioids doses as a response to increasing pain reports can occur when patients use these medications to treat a sleep disorder, anxiety, depression, or other nonpain conditions. Opioids may make patients sleepy and may calm an anxious patient. Insomnia and anxiety may make pain worse as well. Despite the demonstrated efficacy in these other conditions, opioids should not be increased. The appropriate treatment is to address the underlying problem(s) and treat the underlying stress, depression, or insomnia without escalating the opioid dose.

Clinical differentiation includes absence of history, examination, and investigations that suggest increase pathology, pain flare, tolerance, addiction, and psychological stressors. In addition, it is helpful to discover positive indicators of OIH including altered quality of pain, allodynia, extension of pain localization beyond the original site.

## Pathophysiology—Why Does It Happen

It is not fully understood in humans the prevalence of OIH or even the cause. There has been one prospective study in six opioid-naive chronic pain patients demonstrating the development of OIH after one month of oral morphine using quantitative sensory pain measurements (8).

However, in other animal models, there has been progress in elucidating mechanisms present in OIH. The body has methods of transmitting nociceptive signals through receptors in peripheral tissues and pathways that end in centers in the brain that interpret the incoming message. These pathways initiate pain through neurotransmitters such as prostaglandins initiating pain transmission in osteoarthritis. Pain can be augmented (pronociceptive) by increasing the ascending signaling through a variety of transmitters including capsaicin (extract from chili peppers) and excitatory amino acid such as glutamate and its derivative *N*-methyl-D-asparate (NMDA). Pain can be dampened (antinociceptive) by increasing the descending signaling through a variety of transmitters including serotonin and norepinephrine. Abnormalities in ascending and descending pathways may be present in OIH.

NMDA receptors have been implicated in opioid tolerance and OIH (9). NMDA receptors are not involved in acute pain transmission but with repeated pain signaling, persistent pain can develop through NMDA-receptor mechanisms. Descending pathways are frequently inhibitory, lowering pain levels, but changes occur with persistent pain and exposure to opioids stimulating descending pain facilitation mechanisms (10).

Opioids are principally antinociceptive affecting pain transmission such as at the dorsal horn of the spinal cord. In the opioid-tolerant state, however, an anti-opioid system is upregulated, resulting in an increased pronociceptive activity under basal conditions. Further repeated opioid administration causes more upregulation of the anti-opioid system increasing pain levels (11).

Opioid metabolites may also play a role in increasing pain transmission. Morphine is metabolized into several compounds including morphine-3-glucuronide that is known to cause neuroexcitation and increase pain signaling (12).

Additional information on the pathophysiology and the cellular mechanisms of OIH can be found in other chapters in this book.

## Consequences of Ignoring the Problem—Why Important to Me

When a patient presents in pain, discovery of the underlying pathology is vital. Once this anatomy or neurochemistry is found, treatment can be targeted at the cause. Patients frequently get opioids during the initial workup in order to deal with the suffering while pathology is detected. When the underlying cause cannot be found or the treatments are ineffective, continued symptomatic treatment is still imperative. Patients become reliant on the opioid to maintain function, continue to work, and enjoy social activities.

The absolute principle in all of medical care is *primum non nocere* (first, do no harm). If we are trying to treat the suffering, lessen pain, improve function and overall quality of life, then it is essential to know if the treatment is making patients better or worse. Patients themselves are not aware of OIH, only that the opioid seems to be improving the pain. Hyperalgesia then could be causing harm and we must be able to distinguish the difference in order to give the best, most appropriate care.

## Management—What Can I Do About It

When confronted with a patient who is not improving on opioid management or has worsening pain, the differential described earlier should be entertained. Not infrequently, the exact cause may be unclear and the patient may resist a change in therapy including tapering off the opioid. If unsure about the role of tolerance confronting unrelieved pain, the best practical step would be an opioid dose escalation, using the same opioid as before. If the patient's pain improves, but not just transiently, then this is likely to be primarily tolerance. If it worsens or changes character, it is likely to be due to OIH.

Another reasonable approach in such situations includes reduction of opioid dose. Considerable clinical confidence is required to reduce opioid doses in patients experiencing severe pain. During this time, instituting multimodal analgesia with adjuvant therapies as tricyclic antidepressants, nonsteroidal anti inflammatories, NMDA-receptor antagonists, or regional techniques may help the initial increase pain due to opioid tapering. The NMDA receptor may have a central role in the pathophysiology of OIH. Multiple successful trials have demonstrated the efficacy of NMDA-receptor antagonists such as ketamine and dextromethorphan in OIH (13–15).

Opioids have effects at a variety of receptors ($\mu$, $\kappa$, $\delta$), and different opioids not only act differently on these receptors but also have different affinities for the subclasses of the same receptor (16). Accordingly, their propensity to induce the pronociceptive system (and hence hyperalgesia) also differs from one opioid to another. Because of this and known genetic variability, opioid rotation has been successfully used in OIH. Several reports have shown that opioid rotation to methadone significantly improved or resolved suspected OIH (17,18). More discussion on opioid rotation and adjuvant medications can be found in other chapters in the book.

## Recognizing Limitations and Need for Referral—When Do I Need Help

In a busy practice with limited time and difficult clinical decisions, some providers refer any patient using long-term opioid therapy to a specialist. Making the diagnosis of OIH can be tricky even for the experienced clinician. For many patients, answers to the questions asked earlier lead to a management strategy that will often be successful.

First, if the underlying pathology is worsening, treat the pathology. Second, if there are psychosocial comorbidites including anxiety, depression, and substance abuse driving the increased pain complaint, treat the comorbidity. Third, if the increased pain gets better with increasing doses of opioid, it is likely to be opioid tolerance and the treatment should be continued. If the increased pain gets worsen with increasing doses of opioid and is accompanied with a different distribution and character, it is likely to be OIH and opioid rotation, tapering, and adjuvant medications may be helpful.

When this simple approach does not yield the expected outcome, referral to a pain specialist is in order. Continuing the analgesic when the opioid is aggravating the painful condition is ill advised. Tapering the dose or rotation to a different opioid can improve comfort and function.

## CONCLUSIONS

Persistent pain, a highly prevalent condition in the United States, has a significant impact on our health and productivity as a society as well as on our medical and financial resources. Primary care is the most appropriate setting for the management of patients with chronic pain because of the mutual understanding that results from a long-standing physician-patient relationship. The barriers to managing persistent pain are significant but not insurmountable.

Persistent pain is similar to other chronic illnesses but also has many differences making management complicated and difficult in the busy primary care office. OIH is another wrinkle in a complex treatment environment. Due to the vast number of patients experiencing pain and exposed to opioids for long periods of time, OIH will become better recognized and treated. It is vital that the diagnosis be entertained early, at the primary care level, and that intervention also occur just as rapidly. This should stop ever increasing opioid escalation or the perception that opioids are no longer effective. The primary care provider should be the first line in treatment of OIH, but this will only occur with education, simple treatment guidelines, easily understood outcome measures, and a community of pain experts willing to guide us along in the development of this new knowledge.

## REFERENCES

1. O'Rorke JE, Chen I, Genao I, et al. Physicians' comfort in caring for patients with chronic nonmalignant pain. Am J Med Sci 2007; 333:93–100.
2. IMS NPA Health Data 2006.
3. Ballantyne JC, Mao J. Opioid therapy for chronic pain. N Engl J Med 2003; 349:1943–1953.
4. Annals of Family Medicine 2004; 2(1).

5. Gallup, Inc. Pain in America: Highlights from a Gallup Survey. June 9, 1999, Washington, DC.

6. Bostrom BM, Ramberg T, Davis BD, et al. Survey of post-operative patients' pain management. J Nurs Manag 1997; 5:341–349.

7. Dworkin R, Backonja M, Rowbotham M, et al. Advances in neuropathic pain: diagnosis, mechanisms, and treatment recommendations. Arch Neurol 2003; 60:1524–1534.

8. Chu LF, Clark DJ, Angst MS. Opioid tolerance and hyperalgesia in chronic pain patients after one month of oral morphine therapy: a priliminary prospective study. J Pain 2006; 7:43–48.

9. Chu LF, Angst MS, Clark D. Opioid-induced hyperalgesia in humans: molecular mechanism and clinical consderations. Clin J Pain 2008; 24(6):479–496.

10. Ossipov MH, Lai J, King T, et al. Antinociceptive and nociceptive actions of opioids. J Neurobiol 2004; 61:126–148.

11. Chang G, Chen I, Mao J. Opioid tolerance and hyperalgesia. Med Clin North Am 2007; 91:199–211.

12. Hemstapat K, Monteith DR, Smith D, et al. Morphine-3-glucuronide's neuro-excitatory effects are mediated via indirect activation of *N*-methly-D-aspartic acid receptors: mechanistic studies in embryonic cultured hippocampal neurones. Anesth Analg 2003; 97:494–505.

13. Koppert W, Schmelz M. The impact of opioid-induced hyperalgesia for postoperative pain. Best Pract Res Clin Anaesthesiol 2007; 21:65–83.

14. Visser E, Schug SA. The role of ketamine in pain management. Biomed Pharmacother 2006; 60:341–348.

15. Ilkjaer S, Bach LF, Nielsen PA, et al. Effect of preoperative oral dextromethorphan on immediate and late postoperative pain and hyperalgesia after total abdominal hysterectomy. Pain 2000; 86(1–6):19–24.

16. Sukanya M. Opioid-induced hyperalgesia: pathophysiology and clinical implications. J Opoid Manag 2008; 4(3):123–130.

17. Sjogren P. Jensen NH, Jensen TS. Disappearance of morphine-induced hyperalgesia after discontinuing or substituting morphine with other opioid agonists. Pain 1994; 59:313–316.

18. Axelrod DJ, Reville B. Using methadone to treat opioid-induced hyperalgesia and refractory pain. J Opioid Manag 2007; 3:113–114.

# 8

# Managing Opioid-Induced Hyperalgesia in the Perioperative Period

**Matthew Crooks**

*Department of Anesthesiology, Pain Management Division, David Geffen School of Medicine at UCLA, Los Angeles, California, U.S.A.*

**Steven P. Cohen**

*Pain Management Division, Johns Hopkins School of Medicine, Baltimore, Maryland and Walter Reed Army Medical Center, Washington, D.C., U.S.A.*

## BACKGROUND AND SCOPE

Opioid analgesics have been used for pain relief for thousands of years (1). In modern times, they have been mostly employed to treat acute and cancer-related pain. More recently, their use has expanded to include chronic nonmalignant pain. The consistent, effective analgesia that this drug class provides has established opioids as the gold standard to address moderate to severe pain. As their therapeutic use becomes increasingly common, it is incumbent upon physicians to appropriately manage the potential detrimental effects of them. These effects are particularly relevant in the context of surgical intervention.

The opioid-dependent patient poses special challenges for the anesthesiologist in the peri- and postoperative settings. A patient's regular opioid dose may be inadvertently discontinued prior to starting surgery, leading to the early stages of withdrawal. The patient's baseline opioid dosage should thus be accounted for intraoperatively. Opioid-dependent patients frequently require analgesic doses in excess of the general population for a given surgery, which is usually attributed to opioid tolerance (2–4). Yet despite higher opioid usage, these patients tend to also have higher pain scores in the postoperative period (5,6). The same opioid medications utilized to alleviate a patient's pain may lead to a greater sensitivity to pain, a phenomenon known as opioid-induced hyperalgesia (OIH). This is most likely to occur in patients on long-term opioid therapy, but the phenomenon has also been demonstrated in patients receiving short-term opioids, including those whose first exposure is perioperatively (7–9).

Opioids are currently the second most frequently prescribed medication for chronic pain, behind only nonsteroidal anti-inflammatory drugs (NSAIDs) (10). It is estimated that over 10 million patients in the United States are prescribed opioids in any given week, with over 4 million taking them regularly. In one recent study, the most frequently prescribed opioid was hydrocodone (11). Concurrent with the increased frequency with which opioids are prescribed for noncancer pain, the abuse of prescription opioids has also surged. Addiction occurs in an estimated 10% of patients who receive prescription opioids for pain, and aberrant behaviors are observed in up to 40% of these patients (12–16). Another growing subgroup of patients on opioids are former substance abusers in methadone maintenance programs.

The surgical population may contain a disproportionate percentage of opioid users for several reasons (17). Chronic pain is not only a disease unto itself but also a symptom of disease. These patients therefore generally have a higher prevalence rate of systemic disease and disability than the general population, and can logically be assumed to require surgical intervention more frequently. This may occur in the context of a procedure to correct the root cause of pain itself [e.g., spine surgery, palliative cancer surgery, oncological surgery, and trauma surgery stemming from motor vehicle accidents (MVAs), falls, and violence].

## MECHANISMS

OIH arises from sensitization in the central nervous system. Central sensitization can both initiate pain and potentiate pain that outlasts an initial stimulus. This sensitization is triggered in part by an activation of spinal $N$-methyl-D-aspartic acid (NMDA) receptors mediated by the glutamatergic system. NMDA receptors have been implicated in the wind-up phenomenon that is intimately involved in central sensitivity. Tolerance to the analgesic effects of opioids classically develops from decreasing efficacy in the face of long-term administration. Multiple preclinical and clinical studies have documented that in addition to traditional receptor-based tolerance, the diminished antinociceptive effect of opioids is at least partially due to heightened pronociceptive activity (18–21).

The antinociceptive effects of opioids are activated via peripheral, spinal, and supraspinal opioid receptors of four subtypes: $\mu$, $\delta$, $\kappa$, and ORL-1. Activation of G-proteins triggers the antinociceptive effects by several mechanisms. Neuronal excitability is reduced via membrane hyperpolarization caused by the closing of calcium-gated channels. Release of glutamate and substance P can be inhibited by reducing intracellular cAMP. Descending inhibition in the peri-aqueductal gray matter and rostral ventromedial medulla oblongata inhibits on-type cells activated by painful stimuli, and activates off-type cells (22–24).

Pronociceptive effects of opioid have been characterized as well. The cAMP levels increase with long-term exposure to μ agonists, which in turn leads to an increase in excitatory spinal neurotransmitters, and enhanced activity in the periaqueductal gray and midbrain. μ-opioid receptors trigger protein kinase C-induced activation of NMDA receptors, which in turn results in phosphorylation and inactivation of opioid receptors via a negative feedback loop. Activation of nitric oxide synthesis generates nitric oxide, which reduces the antinociceptive effect of μ agonists. Peptides with pronociceptive characteristics can also be induced by the long-term application of opioids. Direct acting pronociceptive peptides include cholecystokinin (CCK), neuropeptide FF (NPFF), and noci-ceptin (orphanin FQ).

Whereas the symptoms of opioid withdrawal have been appreciated for centuries, more recent evidence suggests that the pronociceptive effects of opioid administration can develop with short-term exposure, even in patients with no previous history of opioid exposure. This may be particularly relevant in the perioperative setting. Studies that relate to this phenomenon can be broadly categorized into three groups: studies involving individuals formerly addicted to opioids and currently treated with methadone; studies involving human volunteers using experimental pain models; and studies undertaken in patients undergoing surgery.

## EXPERIMENTAL STUDIES IN HUMANS

### Methadone Maintenance Patients

A series of studies involving former opioid abusers maintained on methadone have evaluated the concept of OIH (25–28). The standard tools for evaluation typically include either the cold pressor test or an electrical stimulation model, both of which simulate acute pain. Methadone maintenance patients generally demonstrate less tolerance than control subjects with these models. Yet, these studies are not meant to imply a causal relationship. Although one hypothesis is that methadone maintenance is causally related to relative pain intolerance, an alternative explanation is that a preexisting intolerance to pain increases the risk of these individuals for opioid abuse.

### Human Volunteers

Experiments aimed at evaluating OIH in human subjects typically employ short-term infusions of opioids, and thus may be considered more indicative of "surgical context." Peterson et al. (29) studied the response to capsaicin and heat-evoked hyperalgesia in 14 opioid-naive patients who received a remifentanil

infusion. Before and during the second rekindling of sensitization, either remifentanil at 0.1 µg/kg/min or saline was infused. Whereas remifentanil reduced the
areas of thermal pain and secondary hyperalgesia during the opioid infusion, these
indices returned to near baseline 30 minutes after the infusion was stopped. This
compared to around 80% of baseline in the placebo group.

Hood et al. (30) employed a heat-capsaicin sensitization model to study
OIH in 10 opioid-naive subjects. A remifentanil infusion was titrated to achieve
more than 50% pain reduction. During the remifentanil infusion, the areas of
allodynia and hyperalgesia were reduced. But after cessation of the infusion, the
areas of secondary hyperalgesia and allodynia increased significantly in the 200-
to 240-minute period, and remained so over 24 hours. Interestingly, the pain
response in regular skin was not different before and after the opioid infusion.
These findings are consistent with animal studies demonstrating hyperalgesia
associated with withdrawal.

The role of the NMDA receptor system in mediating the hyperalgesic
response to opioids was studied by Angst et al. (31) in a double-blind, placebo-
controlled crossover study. After creating an area of mechanical hyperalgesia
on the arm, 10 opioid-naive subjects received the following four infusions on
4 different days: ketamine plus saline, ketamine plus remifentanil, remifentanil
plus saline, or saline plus saline. The area of skin already rendered hyperalgesic
to mechanical stimuli extended significantly after infusion of remifentanil alone,
with normal skin exhibiting no difference in the response to heat stimuli before
and after the remifentanil infusion. Co-infusion of the NMDA antagonist ketamine with remifentanil prevented the expansion of hyperalgesia observed after
remifentanil alone. The infusion of ketamine alone exerted antihyperalgesic and
analgesic effects, making it impossible to discern whether remifentanil-induced
OIH was prevented or merely masked by the analgesic properties of ketamine.
Complicating matters is that not all studies have demonstrated that concurrent
ketamine administration can abolish OIH (32). One possible explanation for the
discrepancy is that nociceptive input in the "negative studies" was stronger than
in the "positive studies." Subanesthetic ketamine might therefore be less effective in preventing or reversing peripheral sensitization than central sensitization.

Whereas NMDA receptor systems appear to play a role in the propagation
of OIH, other networks also affect the complex phenomenon of hyperalgesia
after opioid exposure. Koppert et al. (33) evaluated the effects of clonidine on
OIH propagation in an elegant experimental model that used high current density
transcutaneous electrical stimulation to induce acute pain and secondary
mechanical hyperalgesia in 13 healthy volunteers. Six separate trials one week
apart were done with infusions of normal saline, remifentanil 0.1 µg/kg/min
alone, ketamine 5 µg/kg/min alone, clonidine 2 µg/kg bolus alone, remifentanil
and ketamine, or remifentanil plus clonidine. Consistent with other studies,
remifentanil infusion alone decreased the area of secondary mechanical hyperalgesia during the time of infusion, but in the postinfusion period increased
hyperalgesia was observed. The addition of ketamine to remifentanil abolished

the increased hyperalgesia observed with remifentanil alone. Interestingly, concurrent ketamine infusion reduced acute pain scores compared with remifentanil alone, but had little effect on pain scores following the infusion. This suggests different mechanisms for anti-analgesia and hyperalgesia. Clonidine demonstrated no anti-analgesic or hyperalgesic characteristics by itself, but did produce synergistic effects when combined with remifentanil. Clonidine is utilized clinically in treatment of opioid withdrawal, and thus may partially mimic opioid receptor activation via hyperpolarization and reduced excitability at dorsal horn neurons.

## Clinical Studies

Studies evaluating opioid consumption and pain scores in patients undergoing surgery also suggest that OIH may be clinically relevant. In a study by Guignard et al. (7) done in patients undergoing abdominal surgery, subjects were randomized to receive either 0.5 MAC desflurane plus remifentanil infusion titrated to autonomic responses (remifentanil group) or a constant remifentanil infusion plus desflurane titrated to autonomic responses (desflurane group). Both groups received the same dose of morphine 40 minutes before the end of surgery, and subsequent morphine requirement and pain scores were measured in the first 24 hours postoperatively. The remifentanil group was noted to have significantly higher pain scores despite earlier and higher requirements for morphine than the desflurane group. Although opioid tolerance may explain the findings of increased morphine requirements in the remifentanil group postoperatively, the increased pain scores in combination with increased morphine consumption point more in the direction of OIH, or more precisely, a mixed state of tolerance and OIH.

The effects of opioid dosing on pain scores and analgesic requirements were studied by Chia et al. (8) in a clinical trial undertaken in patients undergoing total abdominal hysterectomy. Sixty patients were randomized to receive either 15 µg/kg preoperatively followed by a fentanyl infusion of 100 µg/hr plus halothane anesthesia (high-dose fentanyl), or 1 µg/kg of fentanyl preoperatively plus halothane alone intraoperatively (low dose). Postoperative pain scores in 4-hour increments and fentanyl consumption were measured for the first 16 hours after surgery. Pain scores in the high-dose fentanyl group were greater at four and eight hours following surgery than in the control group despite up to 50% higher fentanyl requirements. Although not specifically addressed by the authors, these findings suggest a state of hyperalgesia in parallel with opioid tolerance.

A study by Cooper et al. (34) examined 60 patients undergoing cesarean section that were randomized to receive intrathecal bupivacaine plus or minus intrathecal fentanyl. Pain scores and intravenous patient-controlled analgesia (PCA) morphine requirements were similar in the two groups up to 6 hours after delivery, but between 6 and 24 hours after delivery, morphine requirements were 63% higher in the intrathecal fentanyl group.

In contrast to the aforementioned studies, a prospective trial by Cortinez et al. (35) found no evidence of remifentanil-induced acute opioid tolerance. Sixty patients undergoing gynecological surgery were randomized to receive either remifentanil 0.25 µg/kg/min plus sevoflurane mixed with 50% nitrous oxide, or sevoflurane and nitrous oxide alone. The authors found no difference in either pain scores or morphine consumption between groups in the first 24 hours postoperatively. These results are noteworthy in that they found no evidence of acute opioid tolerance in a similar patient population in whom Guignard et al. (7) did observe this phenomenon. One explanation for the difference is that acute opioid tolerance may be dose-dependent, as the Cortinez group employed a remifentanil infusion rate more than three times higher than that used in the Guignard study.

Several opioid treatment variables can influence pain perception and tolerance in response to clinical stimuli. Cohen et al. (6) developed a clinically relevant treatment model to measure the effects opioid dose and treatment duration have on pain response. Prior to a variety of different interventional nerve blocks, patients were given a standard subcutaneous local anesthetic injection with 1 mL of lidocaine. Pain and unpleasantness scores were then recorded prior to further superficial anesthesia administration. A small but consistent statistically significant correlation was found between opioid dose and both pain and unpleasantness. This relationship was maintained across age, gender, and site of procedure. A similar relationship was noted for duration of opioid treatment and both outcome variables.

In the Cohen et al. (6) study, patients on opioids tended to report slightly higher pleasantness scores than pain scores. In the discussion, the authors offered several possible explanations for this phenomenon. One postulated that the phenomenon of OIH exerts a greater effect on pain processing (e.g., cognitive and emotional components) and modulation than it does on transduction and transmission. A second hypothesis proposed that unpleasantness scores might be a more reliable indicator of pain tolerance, whereas pain scores better reflect nociceptive threshold. This is consistent with experimental studies demonstrating pain tolerance to be a more reliable barometer of OIH than pain rating scales (26,36).

## PERIOPERATIVE MANAGEMENT

### Opioid Management

The perioperative management of patients taking chronic opioids is a task fraught with peril. Whereas most clinical studies investigating OIH involved healthy, opioid-naive subjects, the clinical scenario whereby OIH is encountered is distinctly different. In the perioperative context, most patients with OIH will be maintained on opioids for periods ranging from months to decades, with a large percentage exhibiting signs of psychological dependence. Patients on chronic opioid therapy demonstrate tolerance not only to opioids, but also to other central nervous system depressants (i.e., benzodiazepines), as well as intolerance to pain.

Strategies to address postsurgical pain should begin in the preoperative period, and may employ a number of agents and techniques. Critical to addressing OIH is identifying the patient at risk for it. This starts with a thorough history and physical exam, including cataloging the patient's medication list and social history. Emphasis should be placed on prior surgical procedures, with both patient report and previous anesthesia and hospital records warranting consideration. The anesthesiologist must understand the social stigma that comes with labels such as "opioid user" or "abuser," and sensitivity to these issues is integral to building a trusting relationship. Even medical terms such as "dependence" and "tolerance" can have negative connotations to a layperson. Among the various subgroups that fall into this "high-risk" category are patients on long-term opioid treatment for cancer or nonmalignant chronic pain; the opioid abuser of either illicit or prescription drugs; and the former opioid abuser who is maintained on methadone. Clinically, it is impossible to distinguish the contribution of OIH to tolerance without a trial of drug weaning.

An important step in managing the opioid-dependent surgical patient is instructing them to take their morning opioid dose. This should enable basal opioid requirements to be met in patients maintained on long-acting preparations, since most sustained-release preparations provide 12 to 24 hours of analgesia. Like methadone, sustained-release opioids should be restarted as soon as the patient is able to tolerate oral medications. Transdermal fentanyl patches can be maintained without interruption throughout the perioperative period, though hyperthermia in the operating room can speed the absorption. Patients should be advised before surgery to place the patch on an area of the body that would not interfere with surgery. Other analgesics, including NSAIDs, should be taken the day of surgery unless contraindicated (i.e., for certain orthopedic procedures).

For patients who fail to take their morning short-acting opioid, an equivalent loading dose can be given pre- or intraoperatively in parenteral form. Intravenous, epidural, and intrathecal opioid infusions can and should be continued. Opioid antagonists should be avoided in the opioid-dependent patient, and medications such as naltrexone, a long-acting opioid antagonist, should be discontinued. In patients who continue to take opioid antagonists, caution must be exercised since upregulation of $\mu$ receptors can result in exquisite sensitivity to opioids.

Mixed agonist-antagonists such as buprenorphine may be less likely to cause OIH than pure agonists. Although some experts maintain they should be continued throughout the perioperative period (37), their ceiling effect and high receptor affinity may potentially result in inadequate postoperative pain control (i.e., supplemental opioids will not easily displace buprenorphine from opioid receptors). In opioid-exposed patients anticipated to have a challenging postoperative pain course (i.e., those with a previous history of inadequate pain control or who are scheduled for a painful surgery such as thoracotomy), it may be prudent to discontinue buprenorphine at least three days prior to the operation and restart it when postoperative pain is well controlled.

Opioids may need to be liberally utilized intraoperatively to account for μ-opioid receptor down regulation. While there is no standard calculation for how much requirements increase, it is estimated that opioid-tolerant patients require between 50% and greater than 100% higher doses than opioid-naive patients (38,39). This is typically either "front loaded" with the full dose prior to induction or divided, with half given before induction and the remainder titrated in during surgery. It is important to remember that pain typically increases after terminating the infusion of short-acting opioids such as remifentanil. This effect may be less pronounced when the opioid duration of action is longer (22). Postoperatively, the patient can be transitioned to PCA when pain and vital signs are stable. Although there has been controversy in the past over the worsening or recurrence of addictive behavior pattern in active or recovering addicts receiving perioperative opioids, the consensus now holds that pain complaints should be treated seriously in these patients. Basal opioid requirements should be met with long-acting opioids, or in patients who remain nihil per os, with a basal PCA infusion calculated from the preoperative opioid dose. Incident or breakthrough pain should be addressed with sliding scale short-acting opioids, either in the form of pills or demand-dose PCA. There is some evidence that combining low-dose ketamine with morphine can enhance pain relief while reducing overall opioid requirements (40,41).

Methadone is a frequently prescribed synthetic opioid that acts via several other receptor systems besides μ receptors. These actions include antagonism at the NMDA receptor, and inhibition of serotonin and norepinephrine reuptake. The methadone user poses unique challenges from a pharmacological perspective. There is significant interindividual variability in pharmacokinetics, with variable degrees of metabolism by the cytochrome p450 system. This results in a long and unpredictable half-life. There is extensive interaction with other medications, and widely disparate figures cited for equianalgesic potency. Methadone is greater than 80% bound to plasma proteins, mostly α-1 acid glycoprotein, whose plasma level fluctuates with conditions such as stress, disease, chronic opioid use, and consumption of other medications. Because of its long elimination half-life and potential for accumulation, aggressive dose titration can lead to overdose.

It is recommended that these patients be seen in consult with an anesthesiologist preoperatively, take their normal methadone dose the morning of surgery, bring their methadone to the surgicenter or hospital (if not readily available), and resume dosing per routine as soon as the patient tolerates oral intake. In the interim, an alternative analgesic method can be employed, such as PCA, or when possible, regional anesthesia. If regional anesthesia is utilized, a reduced dose of opioids (i.e., >25% of the preoperative dose) must still be

**Table 1** Equianalgesic Opioid Conversion Chart

Morphine, 30 mg
Oxycodone, 20 mg
Hydrocodone, 30 mg
Hydromorphone, 6 mg
Methadone, 4 mg[a]
Meperidine, 300 mg
Codeine, 200 mg
Propoxyphene, 200 mg
Oxymorphone, 10 mg
Transdermal fentanyl, 12.5 μg/hr
Oral transmucosal fentanyl, 400–600 μg
Intrathecal morphine, 0.1 mg

All medications per os unless otherwise specified.
[a]The conversion of methadone to other opioids or vice versa is dose-dependent
(i.e., the higher the dose of opioid, the greater the conversion ratio).

administered in order to prevent withdrawal. An alternative treatment plan might entail the use of clonidine. When converting from methadone to another opioid, a conservative strategy should be employed, keeping in mind incomplete cross-tolerance and varied oral bioavailability (Table 1).

## Preemptive Analgesia

Persistent nociceptive input from peripheral neurons through the perioperative period can induce central sensitization via wind-up phenomena. The result of this central sensitization is prolonged pain and hypersensitivity beyond the period of the initial surgical insult. Peripheral input can be interrupted by NSAIDs, local anesthetics, anticonvulsants, and opioids (42,43). Preemptive analgesia, or the prevention of wind-up stemming from a therapeutic intervention prior to incision that modulates peripheral stimulation, has been the focus of much study. Up to now, the evidence for quantitative success in pain preemption has been equivocal, with clinical studies failing to consistently demonstrate the promising results observed in animal studies (44).

   This concept has evolved to include the disruption of peripheral stimuli in the preoperative, intraoperative, and postoperative periods. Because nociceptive input continues throughout the perioperative period, the opportunity exists to mitigate windup beyond the time prior to incision. Preemptive analgesia has been described as a treatment initiated before surgical incision that remains operational during the surgical procedure and serves to prevent the establishment of altered sensory processing that amplifies postoperative pain. This was traditionally determined by comparing a preincisional treatment to an identical

**Table 2** Evidence Supporting the Preemptive Effects of Various Types of Surgical Analgesia

| Type of analgesia | Evidence for preemptive effect |
| --- | --- |
| Epidural analgesia | Moderate |
| Local anesthesia | Weak to moderate |
| NMDA receptor antagonists | Conflicting |
| Nonsteroidal anti-inflammatory drug | Weak to moderate |
| Opioids | Conflicting |
| Gabapentin | Moderate |
| Tricyclic antidepressants | Weak and conflicting |

*Abbreviation*: NMDA, *N*-methyl-D-aspartic acid.

postincisional treatment with regard to their effects on postoperative analgesia and opioid consumption (45,46). On the basis of this model, administering the drug or applying the intervention before the barrage of nociceptive input begins should be more effective at reducing pain and analgesic consumption than after surgery commences (42,46–48). A second approach for evaluating the "preventative effects" of an intervention is to compare a specific intervention to another treatment, a placebo treatment, or no treatment, and evaluate whether the analgesic effect of the intervention exceeds the expected duration of action of the target agent (46). This model is often termed "preventative analgesia," and unlike preemptive analgesia, the intervention being evaluated may or may not be initiated before surgery. For managing the opioid-tolerant patient, both concepts may have clinical relevance (Table 2).

## ADJUVANTS

### NMDA Receptor Antagonists

Given the evidence supporting NMDA receptor sensitization in OIH, it is reasonable to assume that NMDA antagonists can modify this phenomenon in the clinical setting. In fact, NMDA receptor antagonists have received the most attention with respect to preventative analgesia. However, the results have been more promising for some drugs than others. In a meta-analysis evaluating 40 randomized controlled trial studying the effects of preemptive or preventive analgesia of NMDA receptor inhibitors, dextromethorphan (DX) and ketamine were found to have the most significant impact on postoperative pain (42). In 67% of studies employing DX, and 58% of studies of ketamine, either a reduction in pain scores, a decrease in analgesic requirements, or both positive outcomes were reported. Consistent with true preemptive effects, the incurred benefits on postoperative pain perception lasted beyond the duration of action of the NMDA antagonist (five half-lives).

## Ketamine

In animal studies, pretreatment with ketamine has been consistently found to prevent long-lasting, opioid-induced diminution in nociceptive threshold (49,50). In a clinical setting, ketamine may be useful in providing both adjuvant analgesia in the postsurgical opioid-tolerant patient and as a means to attenuate OIH, even at subanalgesic doses (31,33,51,52). Cohen et al. (41) reported managing the pain of a tetraplegic patient with severe, intractable central pain with IV PCA ketamine for almost one year, dramatically decreasing pain levels and allowing a significant reduction in opioids. Yet, while ketamine has been demonstrated to improve pain control and abolish OIH (53–55), no single clinical dosing regimen has been established as superior.

## Dextromethorphan

Dextromethorphan, a noncompetitive, low-affinity NMDA antagonist, is the D-isomer of the codeine analog levorphanol. A weak opioid often found in cough syrup, it has been shown to provide pain relief postoperatively when adminis-tered pre- or perioperatively in studies of pain hypersensitivity (56–59). DX has been well studied with respect to preemptive analgesia (60–64). In controlled studies examining the effect of preoperative DX administration, treatment patients have usually, (60,63,65,66) but not always (67,68) been found to have lower postoperative pain scores and opioid requirements. Despite the promise of NMDA receptor antagonists in the interrupting windup and mitigating OIH, the ideal dosages and treatment parameters have not been determined.

## MEMBRANE STABILIZERS

### Gabapentinoids

Gabapentin, an anticonvulsant shown to be effective in ameliorating neuropathic pain, has been studied to determine its potential role in the reduction of hyperalgesia. Its binding site, the presynaptic α-2 δ-1 subunit of the voltage-gated calcium channel in dorsal root ganglion cells, facilitates pain hypersen-sitivity in neuropathic pain models. Upregulation of this channel has been verified after nerve injury in rats (69). It is thought that gabapentin may partially exert its effects via NMDA receptors by decreasing the release of the excitatory neurotransmitters glutamate and substance P.

Animal studies have demonstrated that systemic and intrathecal gabapentin can prevent OIH (70–72). In a rat model, van Elstraete et al. (73) induced hyperalgesia in rats via fentanyl injection. Whereas preventative administration of gabapentin 30 minutes prior to fentanyl injection did not affect the early analgesic response to fentanyl, it significantly reduced the long-term decrease in nociceptive threshold. In an experimental rat model of acute pancreatitis, intrathecal gabapentin coadministered with low-dose morphine was more effective at reducing visceral pain compared with either therapy alone (74). Intraperitoneal gabapentin has also been demonstrated to inhibit morphine-induced antinociceptive tolerance in experimental animals, perhaps due to its effects on the $\alpha$-2 $\delta$-1 subunit (75).

Studies conducted in humans have generally supported preclinical work. In a double-blind, placebo-controlled study by Dirks et al. (76), 70 patients were randomized to receive either 1200 mg of gabapentin or placebo 1 hour prior to radical mastectomy, followed by PCA morphine for postoperative pain control. The patients receiving gabapentin experienced significantly less pain despite lower morphine requirements than the placebo group, with no increase in side effects. A meta-analysis by Hurley et al. (77) revealed that 12 of 12 randomized trials evaluating preemptive gabapentin before surgery found that it either reduced pain or diminished opioid requirements, with preoperative dosages ranging from 300 to 1200 mg. Pain scores were reduced in the immediate post-operative period and for up to 24 hours postoperatively. A reduction in anxiety has also been reported in patients receiving gabapentin perioperatively (78).

## Other Anticonvulsants

The potential for other adjunct medications to abolish hyperalgesia is less well established. Mexiletine, an oral analog of lidocaine, is a sodium channel blocker that has been shown to reduce hyperalgesia in mice (79) and improve neuro-pathic pain in humans (80,81). Mexiletine was found to be equipotent to gabapentin in reducing analgesic requirements postoperatively when given for 10 days after surgery (82). When given as a single preincisional dose, it has also been documented to reduce postoperative pain (83). Mexiletine's effectiveness in reducing hyperalgesia is controversial, with some studies asserting its benefit in reducing hyperalgesia (84,85), but others refuting this point (86,87).

Other anticonvulsants have been investigated as a means to abolish hyperalgesia. Lamotrigine has been found to be effective for treatment for peripheral neuropathic and central pain in some studies (88,89), but not all (87,90–92). In an animal model of inflammatory pain, pretreatment with intra-thecal, lamotrigine was found to reduce thermal and mechanical hyperalgesia, suggesting a potential role in preventing OIH (93). Lamotrigine was shown to reduce total analgesic requirements and pain scores when given as a single oral dose preoperatively to patients undergoing transurethral prostatectomy with spinal anesthesia (94).

## Antidepressants

Tricyclic antidepressants have consistently demonstrated efficacy in the treat-ment of chronic neuropathic pain, but have not been widely investigated as adjuvants before surgery. In a preclinical study conducted in rats, Wordliczek et al. (95) found that administering intraperitoneal doxepin 30 minutes before formalin injection significantly elevated the nociceptive threshold after the animals emerged from general anesthesia, but injecting it 240 minutes before or 10 minutes after formalin was given failed to affect the paw-pressure test. When coadministered before morphine, doxepin enhanced the antinociceptive effects of the drug. Levine et al. (96) found that desipramine but not amitriptyline prolonged and enhanced postoperative opioid analgesia when administered for a week before surgery. A similar preemptive effect was found when desipramine was given for only three days before surgery (97). However in a follow-up study, the same group found that preoperative fluoxetine, a serotonergic tricyclic antidepressant, actually attenuated morphine analgesia (98). These findings suggest that drugs that selectively inhibit norepinephrine reuptake may be more effective than serotonin-specific reuptake inhibitors or tertiary amine tricyclic drugs (which preferentially block serotonin reuptake) in providing preventative analgesia. This theory is consistent with preclinical studies demonstrating that desipramine but not fluoxetine can attenuate hyperalgesia in rat models of central sensitization (99).

## Nonsteroidal Anti-Inflammatory Drugs

Prostaglandin inhibitors have been well documented in several reviews and meta-analyses to be effective for postoperative pain control. Their mechanism of action, distinctly different from that of opioids, makes them valuable adjuncts to provide balanced perioperative analgesia. NSAIDs decrease inflammation and pain by inhibiting the synthesis of prostaglandins in the periphery and spinal cord. Both preclinical and clinical studies have demonstrated synergy with opioids. In a rat model, lumiracoxib, codeine, nalbuphine, lumiracoxib-codeine, or lumiracoxib-nalbuphine were injected locally into a formalin-injured paw (100). All treatments produced dose-dependent antinociception; however the NSAID-opioid combination demonstrated a synergistic antinociceptive response of greater than two times the sum of the additive effects of the individual treatments. A similar synergistic antinociceptive response to an NSAID-opioid combination was demonstrated by Miranda et al. (101,102) Interestingly, the individual drugs within classes may dictate the degree NSAID-opioid synergism. For example, different investigators found ibuprofen but neither ketorolac nor aspirin potentiated hydrocodone (103,104).

Nonselective cyclooxygenase inhibitors have been demonstrated to inhibit spinal fusion when administered for postoperative pain control (105). This is thought to be due to an inhibitory effect on osteoblastic activity. The inhibition of fusion, however, may be less of a concern with cyclooxygenase-2 (COX-2) selective inhibitors (106). Although NSAIDs are traditionally thought to act on the periphery, there is emerging evidence that COX-2 inhibitors act centrally as well, and that this central activity can affect nociceptive input, and potentially reduce hyperalgesia (107).

Parecoxib is a parenteral COX-2 inhibitor available outside the United States. Troster et al. (108) found that preventative administration of parecoxib increased the antinociceptive effects of a remifentanil infusion in 15 male volunteers, and significantly diminished the hyperalgesic response after cessation of the infusion. Interestingly, the same effect on hyperalgesia was not found when parecoxib was administered in parallel with remifentanil. Unlike ketamine, parecoxib creates a partial reduction in OIH, not a complete abolition. Nonetheless, these findings suggest a role for prostaglandins in the development of OIH. Acetaminophen, a more centrally acting prostaglandin inhibitor devoid of anti-inflammatory properties, can also reduce intraoperative opioid requirements, and may be used in conjunction with NSAIDs (101).

## Neuraxial Analgesia and Nerve Blocks

Neuraxial techniques may provide a more efficacious means of opioid delivery than parenteral or oral routes (3,109). This allows a greater degree of analgesia postoperatively with a smaller opioid dose, and hence a lower incidence of side effects, than that associated with parenteral administration. In a meta-analysis by Block et al. (110), the authors concluded that epidural analgesia provided superior postoperative analgesia to parenteral opioids, regardless of the epidural agent administered. The addition of local anesthetics and adjuvants such as clonidine can result in further opioid-sparing effects (109,111). Reducing the total opioid dose in the perioperative period may inhibit the development of OIH, which may be a function of both the total dose of opioids and rate of escalation (112–115).

The intrathecal administration of analgesic agents results in an even higher concentration of drug directly delivered to spinal receptors than with epidural dosing. This is advantageous in providing superior efficacy at approximately 1/10th the dose required for epidural delivery. Since epidural administration of lipophilic opioids such as fentanyl result in comparable blood levels to that of intramuscular administration, intrathecal injection generally results in a lower incidence of most opioid-related side effects, though some like pruritis may be higher (116). However, when delivered as a one-time dose, acute withdrawal can occur in opioid-tolerant patients (111,117). Therefore, in patients on high-dose opioids, baseline requirements should be met using oral or intravenous dosing.

Regional analgesia via peripheral nerve block provides a similar opioid-sparing effect when utilized for the appropriate surgical procedure. Placement of an indwelling catheter in proximity to the target nerve(s) can allow for a continuous infusion with extra demand dosing for breakthrough pain in the postoperative period. In a meta-analysis by Richman et al. (118), continuous peripheral nerve block was found to provide superior postoperative analgesia to parenteral or oral opioid analgesia with regard to mean and maximum pain scores and analgesic-related side effects. The addition of clonidine to the local anesthetic mixture can further enhance the ensuing pain relief and opioid-sparing effects (119). Unlike neuraxial analgesia, peripheral nerve blockade is not contraindicated in patients receiving anticoagulation therapy, or with coagulopathy or thrombocytopenia. However, the same caveats apply with respect to avoiding opioid withdrawal in patients taking high baseline doses.

## CONCLUSIONS

As our population ages, chronic pain becomes more prevalent, and aesthetic, curative, and palliative operations become more commonplace, the ability to successfully manage the surgical patient on high-dose opioids will only become more critical. Opioid-tolerant patients pose several unique challenges to perioperative physicians, with OIH being one of the principal ones. Several tools are available to control pain and minimize side effects in patients with suspected OIH, including regional anesthesia, rational polypharmacy, and preemptive analgesia. More studies are needed to better identify OIH and distinguish it from traditional receptor-based tolerance, gain a better appreciation of the scope of the problem, and develop effective means to manage it.

## REFERENCES

1. Blum RH. A history of opium. In: Blum RH, ed. Society and Drugs. San Francisco, CA: Jossey-Bass Inc., 1969.
2. Peng PW, Tumber PS, Gourlay, D. Perioperative pain management of patients on methadone therapy. Can J Anesth 2005; 52:513–523.
3. Mitra S, Sinatra MS. Perioperative management of acute pain in the opioid dependent patient. Anesthesiology 2004; 101:212–227.
4. Carroll IR, Angst MS, Clark JD. Management of pain in patients chronically consuming opioids. Reg Anesth Pain Med 2004; 29:576–591.
5. Seymour RA, Rawlins MD, Rowell FJ. The lancet—Saturday 26 June 1982. Lancet 1982; 1:1425–1426.
6. Cohen SP, Christo PJ, Wang S, et al. The effect of opioid dose and treatment duration on the perception of a painful standardized clinical stimulus. Reg Anesth Pain Med 2008; 33:199–206.
7. Guignard B, Bossard AE, Coste C, et al. Intraoperative remifentanil increases postoperative pain and morphine requirement. Anesthesiology 2000; 93:409–417.
8. Chia YY, Liu K, Wang JJ, et al. Intraoperative high dose fentanyl induces postoperative fentanyl tolerance. Can J Anesth 1999; 46(9):872–877.
9. Cooper DW, Lindsay SL, Ryall DM, et al. Does intrathecal fentanyl produce acute cross-tolerance to i.v. morphine? Br J Anaesth 1997; 78:311–313.
10. Clark JD. Chronic pain prevalence and analgesic prescribing in a general medical population. J Symptom Manage 2002; 23:131–137.
11. Kelly JP, Cook SF, Kaufman DW, et al. Prevalence and characteristics of opioid use in the US adult population. Pain 2008; 138:507–513.
12. Cohen SP, Raja SN. The middle way: a practical approach to prescribing opioids. Nat Clin Pract Neurol 2006; 2:580–581.

13. Katz NP, Sherburne S, Beach M, et al. Behavioral monitoring and urine toxicology testing in patients receiving long-term opioid therapy. Anesth Analg 2003; 97: 1097–1102.

14. Kirsh KL, Whitcomb LA, Donaghy K, et al. Abuse and addiction issues in medically ill patients with pain: attempts at clarification of terms and empirical study. Clin J Pain 2002; 18(suppl 4):S52–S60.

15. Martell BA, O'Connor PG, Kerns RD, et al. Systematic review: opioid treatment for chronic back pain: prevalence, efficacy, and association with addiction. Ann Intern Med 2007; 146:116–127.

16. Miotto MD, Compton P, Ling W, et al. Diagnosing addictive disease in chronic pain patients. Psychosomatics 1996; 3:223–235.

17. Walid MS, Hyer L, Ajjan M, et al. Prevalence of opioid dependence in spine surgery patients and correlation with length of stay. J Opioid Manage 2007; 3:127–128, 130–132.

18. Celerier E, Laulin J, Larcher A, et al. Evidence for opiate activated NMDA processes masking opiate analgesia in rats. Brain Res 1999; 847:18–25.

19. Colpaert FC. System theory of pain and of opiate analgesia: no tolerance to opiates. Pharmacol Rev 1996; 48:355–402.

20. Ossipov MH, Lai J, Vanderah TW, et al. Induction of pain facilitation by sustained opioid exposure: relationship to opioid antinociceptive tolerance. Life Sci 2003; 73:783–800.

21. Simonnet G, Rivat C. Opioid induced hyperalgesia: abnormal or normal pain. Neuroreport 2003; 14:1–7.

22. Koppert W, Schmelz M. The impact of opioid induced hyperalgesia for postoperative pain. Best Pract Res Clin Anaesthesiol 2007; 21:65–83.

23. Heinricher MM, Morgan MM, Fields HL. Direct and indirect actions of morphine on medullary neurons that modulate nociception. Neuroscience 1992; 48:533–543.

24. Heinricher MM, Morgan MM, Fields HL. Disinhibition of off-cells and antinociception produced by an opioid action within the rostral ventromedial medulla. Neuroscience 1994; 63:279–288.

25. Doverty M, White JM, Somogyi AA, et al. Hyperalgesic responses in methadone maintenance patients. Pain 2001; 90:91–96.

26. Doverty M, Somogyi AA, White JM, et al. Methadone maintenance patients are cross-tolerant to the antinociceptive effects of morphine. Pain 2001; 93:155–163.

27. Compton P, Charuvastra VC, Ling W. Pain intolerance in opiate-maintained former opiate addicts: effect of long acting maintenance agent. Drug Alcohol Depend 2001; 63:139–146.

28. Compton P, Charuvastra VC, Kintaudi K, et al. Pain responses in methadone-maintained opiate abusers. J Pain Symptom Manage 2000; 20:237–245.

29. Peterson KL, Jones B, Segredo V, et al. Effect of remifentanil on pain and secondary hyperalgesia associated with the heat-capsaicin sensitization model in healthy volunteers. Anesthesiology 2001; 94:15–20.

30. Hood DD, Curry R, Eisenrach JC. Intravenous remifentanil produces withdrawal hyperalgesia in volunteers with capsaicin-induced hyperalgesia. Anesth Analg 2003; 97:810–815.

31. Angst MS, Koppert W, Pahl I, et al. Short term infusion of the mu opioid agonist remifentanil in humans causes hyperalgesia during withdrawal. Pain 2003; 106: 49–57.

32. Luginbuhl M, Gerber A, Schnider TW, et al. Modulation of remifentanil-induced analgesia, hyperalgesia, and tolerance by small dose ketamine in humans. Anesth Analg 2003; 96:726–732.

33. Koppert W, Sittl R, Scheuber K, et al. Differential modulation of remifentanil-induced analgesia and postinfusion hyperalgesia by S-ketamine and clonidine in humans. Anesthesiology 2003; 99:152–159.

34. Cooper DW, Lindsay SL, Ryall DM, et al. Does intrathecal fentanyl produce acute cross-tolerance to i.v. morphine? Br J Anaesth 2000; 85:807–808.

35. Cortinez LI, Brandes V, Munoz HR, et al. No clinical evidence of acute opioid tolerance after remifentanil-based anaesthesia. Br J Anaesth 2001; 87:866–869.

36. Pud D, Cohen D, Lawental E, et al. Opioids and abnormal pain perception: new evidence from a study of chronic opioid addicts and healthy subjects. Drug Alcohol Depend 2006; 82:218–223.

37. Roberts DM, Meyer-Whitting M. High-dose buprenorphine: perioperative precautions and management strategies. Anaesth Intensive Care 2005; 33:469–476.

38. Saberski L. Postoperative pain management for the patient with chronic pain. In: Sinatra RS, Hord AH, Ginsburg B, et al., eds. Acute Pain: Mechanisms and Management. St. Louis, MO: Mosby Yearbook, 1992:422–431.

39. de Leon-Casasola OA. Cellular mechanisms of opioid tolerance and the clinical approach to the opioid tolerant patient in the post-operative period. Best Pract Res Clin Anaesthesiol 2002; 16:521–525.

40. Haller G, Waeber JL, Infante NK, et al. Ketamine combined with morphine for the management of pain in an opioid addict. Anesthesiology 2002; 96:1265–1266.

41. Cohen SP, DeJesus M. Ketamine patient-controlled analgesia for dysesthetic central pain. Spinal Cord 2004; 42:425–428.

42. McCartney CJ, Sinha A, Katz J. A qualitative systematic review of the role of *N*-methyl D-aspartate antagonists in preventive analgesia. Anesth Analg 2004; 98:1385–1400.

43. Reuben SS, Buvanendran A. Preventing the development of chronic pain after orthopaedic surgery with preventive multimodal analgesic techniques. J Bone Joint Surg (Am) 2007; 89:1343–1358.

44. Grape S, Tramèr MR. Do we need preemptive analgesia for the treatment of postoperative pain? Best Pract Res Clin Anaesthesiol 2007; 21:51–63.

45. Dahl JB, Møiniche S. Pre-emptive analgesia. Br Med Bull 2004; 71:13–27.

46. Kissin, I. Preemptive analgesia at the crossroad. Anesth Analg 2005; 100:754–756.

47. Katz J, McCartney CJ. Current status of preemptive analgesia. Curr Opin Anaesthesiol 2002; 15:435–441.

48. Katz J. Timing of treatment and pre-emptive analgesia. In: Rice A, Warfield C, Justins D, et al, eds. Clinical Pain Management. Vol 1: Acute Pain. London: Arnold, 2003:113–163.

49. Laulin JP, Maurette P, Corcuff JB, et al. The role of ketamine in preventing fentanyl-induced hyperalgesia and subsequent acute morphine tolerance. Anesth Analg 2002; 94:1263–1269.

50. Celerier E, Rivat C, Jun Y, et al. Long-lasting hyperalgesia induced by fentanyl in rats: preventative effect of ketamine. Anesthesiology 2000; 92:465–472.

51. Menigaux C, Guignard B, Fletcher D, et al. Intraoperative small dose ketamine enhances analgesia after outpatient knee arthroscopy. Anesth Analg 2001; 93: 606–612.

52. De Kock M, Lavand'homme P, Waterloos H. 'Balanced analgesia' in the perioperative period: is there a place for ketamine? Pain 2001; 92:373–380.

53. Trujillo KA, Akil H. Inhibition of morphine tolerance and dependence by the NMDA-receptor antagonist MK-801. Science 1991; 251:85–87.

54. Clark JL, Kalan GE. Effective treatment of severe cancer pain of the head using low-dose ketamine in an opioid tolerant patient. J Pain Symptom Manage 1995; 10:310–314.

55. Connor DFJ, Muir A. Balanced analgesia for the management of pain associated with multiple fractured ribs in an opioid addict. Anaesth Intensive Care 1998; 26:459–460.

56. Wu G-T, Yu J-C, Yeh C-C, et al. Preincisional dextromethorphan treatment decreases postoperative pain and opioid requirement after laparoscopic cholecystectomy. Anesth Analg 1999; 88:1331–1334.

57. Dawson GS, Seidman P, Ramadan HH. Improved postoperative pain control in pediatric adenotonsillectomy with dextromethorphan. Laryngoscope 2001; 111: 1223–1226.

58. Moiniche S, Kehlet H, Berg J. A qualitative and quantitative systematic review of preemptive analgesia for postoperative pain relief. Anesthesiology 2002; 96:725–741.

59. Weinbrown AA, Rudick V, Paret G, et al. The role of dextromethorphan in pain control. Can J Anaesth 2000; 47:585–596.

60. Weinbroum AA, Gorodetzky A, Nirkin A, et al. Dextromethorphan for the reduction of immediate and late postoperative pain and morphine consumption in orthopedic oncology patients: a randomized, placebo-controlled, double-blind study. Cancer 2002; 95:1164–1170.

61. Helmy SA, Bali A. The effect of the preemptive use of the NMDA receptor antagonist dextromethorphan on postoperative analgesia requirements. Anesth Analg 2001; 92:739–744.

62. Woolf CJ, Thompson SWN. The induction and maintenance of central sensitization is dependent on $N$-methyl-D-aspartic acid receptor activation: implications for the treatment of post-injury pain hypersensitivity states. Pain 1991; 44:293–299.

63. Weinbroum AA, Gorodezky A, Niv D, et al. Dextromethorphan attenuation of postoperative pain and primary and secondary thermal hyperalgesia. Can J Anaesth 2001; 48:167–174.

64. Woolf CJ, Chong MS. Preemptive analgesia: treating postoperative pain by preventing the establishment of central sensitization. Anesth Analg 1993; 77:362–379.

65. Chia YY, Liu K, Chow LH, et al. The preoperative administration of intravenous dextromethorphan reduces postoperative morphine consumption. Anesth Analg 1999; 89:748–752.

66. Yeh CC, Jao SW, Huh BK, et al. Preincisional dextromethorphan combined with thoracic epidural anesthesia and analgesia improves postoperative pain and bowel function in patients undergoing colonic surgery. Anesth Analg 2005; 100:1384–1389.

67. Rose JB, Cuy R, Cohen DE, et al. Preoperative oral dextromethorphan does not reduce pain or analgesic consumption in children after adenotonsillectomy. Anesth Analg 1999; 88:749–753.

68. Grace RF, Power I, Umedaly H, et al. Preoperative dextromethorphan reduces intraoperative but not postoperative morphine requirements after laparotomy. Anesth Analg 1998; 87:1135–1138.

69. Luo ZD, Chaplan SR, Higuera ES, et al. Upregulation of dorsal root ganglion α2δ calcium channel subunit and its correlation with allodynia in spinal nerve-injured rats. J Neurosci 2001; 21:1868–1875.
70. Hunter JC, Gogas KR, Hedley LR, et al. The effect of novel anti-epileptic drugs in rat experimental models of acute and chronic pain. Eur J Pharmacol 1997; 324: 153–160.
71. Jun JH , Yaksh TL. The effect of intrathecal gabapentin and 3-isobutyl gamma-aminobutyric acid on the hyperalgesia observed after thermal injury in the rat. Anesth Analg 1998; 86:348–354.
72. Jones DL, Sorkin LS. Systemic gabapentin and S(+)-3-isobutyl-gamma amino-butyric acid block secondary hyperalgesia . Brain Res 1998; 810:93–99.
73. van Elstraete AC, Sitbon P, Mazoit JX, et al. Gabapentin prevents delayed and long-lasting hyperalgesia induced by fentanyl in rats. Anesthesiology 2008; 108: 484–494.
74. Smiley MM, Lu Y, Vera-Portocarrero LP, et al. Intrathecal gabapentin enhances the analgesic effects of subtherapeutic dose morphine in a rat experimental pancreatitis model. Anesthesiology 2004; 101:759–765.
75. Gilron I, Biederman J, Jhamandas K, et al. Gabapentin blocks and reverses antinociceptive morphine tolerance in the rat paw-pressure and tail-flick tests. Anesthesioogy 2003; 98:1288–1292.
76. Dirks J, Fredensborg BB, Christensen D, et al. A randomized study of the effects of single-dose gabapentin versus placebo on postoperative pain and morphine consumption after mastectomy. Anesthesiology 2002; 97:560–564.
77. Hurley RW, Cohen SP, Williams KA, et al. The analgesic effect of perioperative gabapentin on postoperative pain: a meta-analysis. Reg Anesth Pain Med 2006; 31:237–247.
78. Menigaux C, Adam F, Guignard B, et al. Preoperative gabapentin decreases anxiety and improves early functional recovery from knee surgery. Anesth Analg 2005; 100:1394–1399.
79. Kamei J, Hitosugi H, Kasuya Y. Effects of mexiletine on formalin-induced nociceptive responses in mice. Res Commun Chem Pathol Pharmacol 1993; 80: 153–162.
80. Dejgard A, Petersen P, Kastrup J. Mexiletine for treatment of chronic painful diabetic neuropathy. Lancet 1988; 1:9–11.
81. Sloan P, Basta M, Storey P, et al. Mexiletine as an adjuvant analgesic for the management of neuropathic cancer pain. Anesth Analg 1999; 89:760–761.
82. Fassoulaki A, Patris K, Sarantopoulos C, et al. The analgesia effect of gabapentin and mexilitine after breast surgery for cancer. Anesth Analg 2002; 95:985–991.
83. Morita H, Higashizawa T, Yuasa H, et al. Evaluation of preincisional mexilitine administration to alleviate postoperative pain. Masui 1998; 47:1311–1314.
84. Joshi SK, Hernandez G, Mikusa JP, et al. Neuroscience 1996; 143:587–596.
85. Klamt JG. Effects of intrathecally administered lamotrigene, a glutamate release inhibitor, on short-and long-term models of hyperalgesia in rats. Anesthsiology 1998; 88:487–494.
86. Wallace MS, Magnson S, Ridgeway B. Efficacy of oral mexiletine for neuropathic pain with allodynia: a double blind, placebo-controlled, cross-over study. Reg Anesth Pain Med 2000; 25:459–467.

87. Silver M, Blum D, Grainger D, et al. Double-blind, placebo-controlled trial of lamotrigine in combination with other medications for neuropathic pain. J Pain Symptom Manage 2007; 34:446–454.
88. Breuer B, Pappagallo M, Knotvola H, et al. A randomized, double-blind, placebo-controlled, two-period, crossover, pilot trial of lamotrigine in patients with central pain due to multiple sclerosis. Clin Ther 2007; 29:2022–2230.
89. Nicolson A, Lewis SA, Smith DF. A prospective analysis of leviteracetam in clinical practice. Neurology 2004; 63:568–570.
90. Pop-Bursui R. Does lamotrigene alleviate the pain in diabetic neuropathy? Pain 2007; 3:424–425.
91. Vink AI, Tuchman M, Safirstein M, et al. Lamotrigine for treatment of pain associated with diabetic neuropathy: results of two randomized, double-blind, placebo-controlled studies. Pain 2007; 128:169–179.
92. Wiffen PJ, Ress J. Lamotrigine for acute and chronic pain. Cochrane Database Syst Rev 2007; 18:CD006044.
93. Lee TH, Wang CJ, Wu PC, et al. The thermal and mechanical anti-hyperalgesic effects of pre- vs. post-intrathecal treatment with lamotrigine in a rat model of inflammatory pain. Life Sci 2002; 70:3039–3047.
94. Bonicalzi V, Canavero S, Cerutti F, et al. Lamotrigine reduces total postoperative analgesic requirement: a randomized double-blind, placebo-controlled pilot study. Surgery 1997; 122:567–570.
95. Wordliczek J, Banach M, Dorazil M, et al. Influence of doxepin used in preemptive analgesia on the nociception in the postoperative period. Experimental and clinical study. Pol J Pharmacol 2001; 53:253–261.
96. Levine JD, Gordon NC, Smith R, et al. Desiprimine enhnaces opioid postoperative analgesia. Pain 1986; 27:45–49.
97. Gordon NC, Heller PH, Gear RW, et al. Temporal factors in the enhancement of morphine analgesia by desiprimine. Pain 1993; 53:273–276.
98. Gordon NC, Heller PH, Gear RW, et al. Interactions between fluoxetine and opiate analgesia for postoperative dental pain. Pain 1994; 58:85–88.
99. Jett MF, McGuirk J, Waligora D, et al. The effects of mexilitine, desipramine, and fluoxetine in rat models involving central sensitization. Pain 1997; 69:161–169.
100. Ortiz MI, Castañeda-Hernández G. Examination of the interaction between peripheral lumiracoxib and opioids on the 1% formalin test in rats. Eur J Pain 2008; 12:233–241.
101. Miranda HF, Puig MM, Dursteler C, et al. Dexketoprofen-induced antinociception in animal models of acute pain: synergy with morphine and paracetamol. Neuropharmacology 2007; 52:291–296.
102. Miranda HF, Prieto JC, Pinardi G. Spinal synergy between nonselective cyclooxygenase inhibitors and morphine antinociception in mice. Brain Res 2005; 1049:165–170.
103. Zelcer S, Kolesnikov Y, Kovalyshyn I, et al. Selective potentiation of opioid analgesia by nonsteroidal anti-inflammatory drugs. Brain Res 2005; 1041:151–156.
104. Kolesnikov YA, Wilson RS, Pasternak GW. The synergistic analgesic interactions between hydrocodone and ibuprofen. Anesth Analg 2003; 97:1721–1723.
105. Glassman SD, Rose SM, Dimar JR, et al. The effect of postoperative nonsteroidal anti-inflammatory drug administration on spinal fusion. Spine 1998; 23:834–838.

106. Long J, Lewis S, Kuklo T, et al. The effect of cyclooxygenase-2 inhibitors on spinal fusion. J Bone Joint Surg (Am) 2004; 84:1763–1768.
107. McCormack K. Non-steroidal anti-inflammatory drugs and spinal nociceptive processing. Pain 1994; 59:9–43.
108. Tröster A, Sittl R, Singler B, et al. Modulation of remifentanil-induced analgesia and postinfusion hyperalgesia by parecoxib in humans. Anesthesiology 2006; 105:1016–1023.
109. Cousins MJ, Veering BT. Epidural neural blockade. In: Cousins MJ, Bridenbaugh PO, eds. Neural Blockade in Clinical Anesthesia and Management of Pain. 3rd ed. Philadelphia, PA: Lippincott–Raven, 1998.
110. Block BM, Liu SS, Rowlingson AJ, et al. Efficacy of postoperative epidural analgesia: a meta-analysis. JAMA 2003; 290:2455–2463.
111. de Leon-Casasola OA, Lema MJ. Epidural bupivacaine/sufentanil therapy for postoperative pain control in patients tolerant to opioid and unresponsive to epidural bupivacaine/morphine. Anesthesiology 1994; 80:303–309.
112. Sjogren P, Jensen NH, Jensen TS. Disappearance of morphine-induced hyperalgesia after discontinuing or substituting morphine with other opioid agonists. Pain 1994; 59:313–316.
113. De Conno F, Caraceni A, Martini C, et al. Hyperalgesia and myoclonus with intrathecal infusion of high-dose morphine. Pain 1991; 47:337–339.
114. Lawlor P, Walker P, Bruera E, et al. Severe opioid toxicity and somatization of psychosocial distress in a cancer patient with a background of chemical dependence. J Pain Symptom Manage 1997; 13:356–361.
115. Sjogren P, Thunedborg LP, Christrup L, et al. Is development of hyperalgesia, allodynia and myoclonus related to morphine metabolism during long-term administration? Six case histories. Acta Anaesthesiol Scand 1998; 42:1070–1075.
116. Cohen SP, Drogovich A. Intrathecal analgesia. Anesthesiol Clin 2007; 25:863–882.
117. de Leon-Casasola OA, Lema MJ. Epidural sufentanil for acute pain control in a patient with extreme opioid dependency. Anesthesiology 1992; 76: 853–856.
118. Richman JM, Liu SS, Courpas G, et al. Does continuous peripheral nerve block provide superior pain control to opioids? A meta-analysis. Anesth Analg 2006; 102:248–257.
119. McCartney CJ, Duggan E, Apatu E. Should we add clonidine to local anesthetic for peripheral nerve blockade? A qualitative systematic review of the literature. Reg Anesth Pain Med 2007; 32:330–338.

# 9

# Role of Ketamine in Managing Opioid-Induced Hyperalgesia

**Yakov Vorobeychik**

*Department of Anesthesiology, Penn State Milton S. Hershey Medical Center,
Penn State College of Medicine, Hershey, Pennsylvania, U.S.A.*

## INTRODUCTION

The role of opioid-induced hyperalgesia (OIH) in clinical situations of reduced opioid responsiveness has been increasingly recognized in chronic pain patients who experience increasing pain despite escalating doses of opioids. A considerable number of studies have investigated the cellular mechanisms of OIH. There is evidence of neuroplasticity occurring in the rostral ventromedial medulla of the brain as well as dorsolateral funiculus of the spinal cord (1–6). Among the neural mechanisms of opioid pronociceptive activity, there is substantial evidence describing the downregulation of glutamate transporters in the spinal cord and activation of $N$-methyl-D-aspartate (NMDA) receptors (7–10). It is not surprising that many researchers and clinicians have focused on investigating the potential role of NMDA receptor antagonists in treatment of OIH. Unfortunately, direct competitive NMDA receptor blockers and high-affinity noncompetitive NMDA antagonists exhibit inadequate therapeutic margins for human use when evaluated in clinical trials (11–14). On the other hand, low affinity blockers were shown to have a better therapeutic index (15). Ketamine appears to be in the middle of the affinity range of noncompetitive NMDA antagonists and is probably the most potent one available for clinical use. This chapter discusses the role of ketamine in treatment of OIH and other conditions such as cancer-related pain.

## MECHANISMS OF ACTION

Ketamine interacts with the NMDA receptor via binding to its phencyclidine site. Because this site is located inside the NMDA receptor-gated ion channel, the binding may take place only when the receptor is activated (16). Some evidence suggests that such a block occurs under tonic NMDA receptor-mediated excitation, which happens under certain pathophysiological conditions, but can be quickly relieved under normal physiological transmission ensuring a more favorable therapeutic profile of this medication (17–19).

It has been hypothesized that the analgesic effect of ketamine may be mediated by the mechanisms other than its interaction with NMDA receptors. Opioid receptors, monoamine reuptake transporters, serotonin, dopamine, and ion channels have all been suggested to have possible implications in ketamine's mechanisms of action (20–24). However, with the exception of $D_2$ dopamine receptors, ketamine's interactions with non-NMDA receptors are significant at anesthetic but not at low analgesic doses. In clinical studies, ketamine produced analgesia at plasma concentrations below 1 $\mu$M, which is relatively selective for NMDA receptors (25). A strong correlation between antihyperalgesic potency and NMDA antagonism has been shown in different competitive and non-competitive NMDA antagonists (18,26). It was also demonstrated that pre-treating healthy volunteers with naloxone did not affect ketamine-induced reduction of secondary hyperalgesia caused by a burn injury (27). Although ketamine binds to $D_2$ dopamine receptors with an affinity similar to its binding to NMDA receptors, which might be related to the mechanism of the ketamine's potential psychotropic effects, pretreatment with the non-selective dopamine receptor antagonist, haloperidol, failed to prevent such effects in humans (28). Therefore, it is unlikely that the central therapeutic analgesic effect of ketamine may be attributed to mechanisms other than NMDA receptor antagonism.

## THERAPEUTIC EFFICACY IN OIH

Both preclinical studies and clinical reports demonstrate the effect of ketamine in OIH. Single dose ketamine pretreatment suppressed the immediate hyperalgesic phase that followed four fentanyl boluses and prevented a fentanyl-elicited long-term decrease of the nociceptive threshold in rats (29). However, subsequent morphine administration restored the long-term hyperalgesia and repeated ketamine infusions were required to obtain a full preventive effect (29). Celerier et al. also evaluated the consequences of four subcutaneous bolus injections of fentanyl in rats and observed an early analgesia (for 2–5 hours) and a later response indicative of hyperalgesia for up to five days. Ketamine pretreatment prevented the development of long-term hyperalgesia (30). Van Elstraete et al.

assessed sensitivity to nociceptive stimuli in rats after an acute intrathecal injection of morphine and observed an early analgesia followed by the delayed hyperalgesia lasting one to two days. A subcutaneous ketamine infusion prior to morphine administration did not affect the early analgesic component but almost completely prevented the delayed hyperalgesia (31). Ketamine was shown not only to improve exaggerated postoperative nociception induced by perioperative opioid use in rats but also to provide better postoperative rehabilitation (32).

Human studies and case reports generally support the experimental data indicating the role of ketamine in prevention and treatment of OIH. Angst et al. in a double-blind, randomized, placebo-controlled, crossover study demonstrated a significant increase of mechanically evoked hyperalgesia in opioid-naive human volunteers within 30 minutes of stopping a 90-minute remifentanil infusion. Coadministration of ketamine abolished the increased hyperalgesia observed after infusion of remifentanil (33). In another recent study, 75 patients undergoing abdominal surgery were randomly divided into three groups. The first group received intraoperative remifentanil at 0.05 µg/kg/min, the second group was given this medication at the large dose of 0.4 µg/kg/min, and the last one received 0.5 mg/kg ketamine in addition to the large dose of intraoperative fentanyl. A large dose of intraoperative fentanyl caused postoperative hyperalgesia that was prevented by the small-dose ketamine infusion (34). Singla et al. reported a case in which a patient with intractable pain due to complex regional pain syndrome (CRPS) was given five boluses of solution containing a total of 75 mg morphine, 300 µg clonidine, and 15 mg bupivacaine administered through an intrathecal pump over just a few hours. Such treatment resulted in opioid toxicity and increase of pain that was attributed by the authors to probable OIH. After the patient was started on an infusion of 100 mg/hr of ketamine along with 2 to 5 mg/hr of midazolam and her intrathecal opioid was changed to sufentanil 50 µg/mL, she became comfortable and continued to have good pain control at the time of discharge (35). Yet, another published case review described a patient with increasingly severe pain with cryoglobulinemia, vasculitis, and cutaneous ulcerations. Her daily opioids, which were started at 45 to 60 mg morphine equivalent dose, underwent a 10-fold increase during a 10-month period resulting in less pain control than she had before the dose escalation. Opioid rotation to methadone helped her obtain adequate pain relief for a few months until only when concomitant cellulitis rekindled her persistent pain. Oral ketamine 20 mg three times a day not only rendered a marked decrease in pain intensity but also afforded substantial reduction of the daily methadone dose (36).

## CLINICAL PROTOCOLS FOR KETAMINE USE

There is no uniformity in ketamine doses and route of administration when used as an analgesic. The following are a few examples of protocols that have been used under various clinical conditions.

Fine administered 0.1 to 0.2 mg/kg ketamine intravenously to treat opioid nonresponsive terminal cancer pain (37). Another protocol suggests slow intravenous boluses of 0.25 to 0.5 mg/kg for patients with similar pain (38).

Good et al. advocated a short-term concurrent use of ketamine, opioid, and anti-inflammatory agent for poorly controlled pain in the palliative care population. Most of the patients in this study received continuous ketamine infusions in the dose range of 100 to 500 mg/day (39).

Okon recommended an intravenous infusion of ketamine at 0.5 mg/kg over four to six hours for intractable opioid-resistant pain. If significant reduction in pain intensity is achieved during this period, the infusion continues at a total dose of 1.5 mg/kg/day for 48 to 72 hours and then is converted 1:1 to a subcutaneous route three times a day. If the pain does not improve, 2 mg/kg of ketamine is infused over the next 12 hours and titrated upwards by 50% to 100% every 24 hours. However, opioid dose reduction must be attempted when the pain is decreased (36).

Jackson et al. successfully used subcutaneous ketamine infusions for three to five days for refractory cancer pain. If the pain persisted, the initial dose of 100 mg/day was gradually escalated up to 500 mg/day. The infusions were discontinued after five days if no noticeable improvement was achieved (40).

While ketamine has a high bioavailability after parenteral administration, its oral bioavailability is only 16.5% (41). Surprisingly, Fitzgibbon et al. reported three patients with difficult pain syndromes whose initial parenteral ketamine at 40 to 60 mg/day was successfully converted to oral ketamine with a 60% to 70% dose reduction. The authors hypothesized that oral ketamine at 1/3 of the parenteral dose is able to maintain the stable levels of its primary active metabolite norketamine (42). Oral ketamine at the dose of 0.5 mg/kg three times daily significantly improved neuropathic pain in cancer patients (43).

Azevedo et al. used transdermal 25 mg/day ketamine patch on 26 patients at the end of gynecological surgery and reported better analgesia compared to the placebo group. No adverse effects were noticed (44). There is substantial preclinical evidence that peripheral NMDA receptors may contribute to neuropathic and inflammatory pain (45,46). In patients with neuropathic pain topical ketamine was found to be effective in some cases; however, its effect may be related either to the blockade of NMDA receptors or to its local anesthetic properties (47–49). Topical ketamine-amitriptyline cream also reduced refractory neuropathic pain in one study (50). Other studies did not confirm its effectiveness in topical form (51).

It has been demonstrated that preservative free epidural ketamine improved analgesia and reduced opioid consumption in children (52,53). Obviously, while there are many different therapeutic protocols for ketamine use, it is undoubted that parenteral infusions afford the quickest and strongest results, whereas oral ketamine causes fewer and less severe side effects. The analgesic efficacy of use of this drug by the transdermal, topical, and intranasal routes still has to be confirmed by more studies.

## KETAMINE USE FOR CANCER PAIN

Ketamine may play a particularly important role in cancer-related opioid-resistant pain treatment. Utilization of high doses of opioid analgesics may lead to the development of opioid unresponsiveness in oncology patients. OIH, pharmacodynamic, pharmacokinetic, and learned tolerance can all cause decreased opioid efficacy in this patient population (54). The notion that opioids may have no "ceiling effect" may have contributed to the use of "megadoses" of these analgesics and, sometimes, to possible opioid toxicity described in such patients. The presence of a neuropathic component in oncological pain also makes it more difficult to manage with opioids (55). Moreover, some patients with intractable cancer pain may develop several of the above-mentioned phenomena during their opioid treatment. In this context, it is noteworthy that OIH, antinociceptive tolerance, and neuropathic pain probably have common mechanisms associated with activation of NMDA receptors by glutamate (54, 56). Hence, administration of the NMDA antagonist ketamine would be very instrumental in overcoming opioid resistance caused by any of these factors.

Many studies published during the last decade showed that low to moderate doses of ketamine significantly improved analgesia in patients with opioid refractory cancer pain. In a randomized, double-blind, placebo-controlled, crossover study, ketamine (0.25 or 0.5 mg/kg) was proven to be effective in cancer patients whose pain was unresponsive to morphine (38). A retrospective review demonstrated an adequate analgesia achieved by intravenous ketamine in 11 of 16 palliative care patients whose pain was previously uncontrolled by opioids. For 13 patients, the ketamine dose ranged from 40 to 50 mg/day, while two patients received 75 mg/day, and one patient received 90 mg/day of ketamine. The authors also reported 25% median opioid dose reduction in their patients (57).

Lossignol et al. successfully used a continuous infusion of a subanesthetic dose of ketamine (1.5 mg/kg/day) in 12 patients with intractable cancer pain and not only attained adequate pain control, but also managed to reduce the total daily dose of morphine by 50% (58). Good et al. have shown that short-term (burst) triple-agent analgesic (ketamine, opioid, and anti-inflammatory agent) administration is effective and safe in palliative care patients in the inpatient setting during episodes of poorly controlled pain (39). The authors established three inclusion criteria for this study: (*i*) unstable pain control, with moderate to severe pain requiring hospitalization; (*ii*) poor response to prior therapy; and (*iii*) high-risk (for poor control) pain mechanisms and syndromes, especially incident and/or neuropathic pain. The starting dose of ketamine was 100 mg/day and the final median dose was 200 mg/day with a range of 100 to 700 mg/day. The median number of days of ketamine use was 5 with a range of 3 to 17 days. To qualify as a responder, the patient had to be pain free or have a 50% or greater reduction in the verbal rating scale score (where 10 = worst imaginable pain and 0 = no pain). In addition, one of the following two criteria had to be fulfilled: (*i*) 50% or greater reduction in the 24-hour opioid use or a 50% or greater reduction in the number of breakthrough doses and (*ii*) improvement in mobility or function. Of the 18 patients, 12 were classified as responders. In yet another study, oral ketamine (0.5 mg/kg three times a day) was used in nine cancer patients experiencing intractable neuropathic pain and taking maximally tolerated doses of morphine, amitriptyline, sodium valproate, or their combination (43). All patients reported initial pain scores of >6 on a 0 to 10 scale. Seven patients exhibited a decrease in the numerical rating score of more than 3; six – within 24 hours of starting oral ketamine, and seven – after 10 days. In dissonance, one systematic review demonstrated lack of suitable randomized trials and insufficient evidence to make recommendation for routine use of ketamine for cancer pain (59). This view remains controversial at this point.

## ADVERSE EFFECTS

Ketamine may cause numerous side effects, such as psych-cognitive or cardio-stimulatory changes, sedation and respiratory depression. Alterations in body image and mood, feelings of unreality, floating sensation, hallucinations, restlessness, vivid dreams, dissociation, insomnia, fatigue, delirium, confusion, and drowsiness are among the cognitive adverse effects described in the literature (60). Increased blood pressure and heart rate are the most common cardiovascular complications (36). NMDA receptor antagonists including ketamine were found to trigger a dose-dependent neurotoxic reaction in the cingulated and retrosplenial cortices of adult rats when administered as a short-term treatment (61). The side effect profile of ketamine has been shown to vary depending on route of administration. Prolonged continuous infusion of intrathecal ketamine was associated with spinal cord vacuolization (62). While oral ketamine produces few adverse effects (63), most of the mentioned side effects have been reported with intravenous and subcutaneous administration of an NMDA antagonist. Moreover, the incidence of side effects with systemic ketamine used in combination with opioids is low and does not differ from controls treated with opioids alone (64). Specifically, hallucinations occur in 7.4%, "pleasant dreams" in 18.3%, nightmares in 4%, and visual disturbance in 6.2% of patients (65). The overall rate of central nervous system adverse effects in patients receiving low-dose ketamine is about 10% (53). It is believed that ketamine may cause psychotomimetic effects by disinhibiting certain excitatory transmitter circuits in the human brain (66). Some drugs, such as benzodiazepines, can restore the inhibition to this circuitry providing a neuroprotective effect and reducing the rate of complications (67). Therefore, concomitant use of benzodiazepines is recommended during ketamine infusion treatment (68). Another class of medications, α-2-adrenergic agonists, may also protect against neurotoxic, psychotomimetic, and cardiostimulatory side effects of ketamine and, in the case of neuropathic pain, exert a synergistic analgesic effect (69–71).

In summary, ketamine is a clinically available NMDA receptor antagonist that has shown its effectiveness in reducing OIH and related clinical conditions.

A number of protocols are available and have been tested in various clinical studies. However, the utility of this agent needs to be balanced with its side effects. Nonetheless, the use of NMDA receptor antagonists such as ketamine should be considered as a clinical approach to managing OIH.

## REFERENCES

1. Vera-Portocarrero LP, Zhang ET, King T, et al. Spinal NK-1 receptor expressing neurons mediate opioid-induced hyperalgesia and antinociceptive tolerance via activation of descending pathways. Pain 2007; 129(1–2):35–45.
2. Gardell LR, Wang R, Burgess SE, et al. Sustained morphine exposure induces a spinal dynorphin-dependent enhancement of excitatory transmitter release from primary afferent fibers. J Neurosci 2002; 22(15):6747–6755.
3. Gardell LR, King T, Ossipov MH, et al. Opioid receptor-mediated hyperalgesia and antinociceptive tolerance induced by sustained opiate delivery. Neurosci Lett 2006; 396(1):44–49.
4. Meng ID, Harasawa I. Chronic morphine exposure increases the proportion of on-cells in the rostral ventromedial medulla in rats. Life Sci 2007; 80(20): 1915–1920.
5. Vera-Portocarrero LP, Zhang ET, Ossipov MH, et al. Descending facilitation from the rostral ventromedial medulla maintains nerve injury-induced central sensitization. Neuroscience 2006; 40(4):1311–1320.
6. Xie JY, Herman DS, Stiller CO, et al. Cholecystokinin in the rostral ventromedial medulla mediates opioid-induced hyperalgesia and antinociceptive tolerance. J Neurosci 2005; 25(2):409–416.
7. Mao J, Sung B, Ji RR, Lim G. Chronic morphine induces downregulation of spinal glutamate transporters: implications in morphine tolerance and abnormal pain sensitivity. J Neurosci 2002; 22(18):8312–8323.
8. Inturrisi CE. The role of $N$-methyl-D-aspartate (NMDA) receptors in pain and morphine tolerance. Minerva Anestesiol 2005; 71(7–8):401–403.
9. Mao J, Mayer DJ. Spinal cord neuroplasticity following repeated opioid exposure and its relation to pathological pain. Ann N Y Acad Sci 2001; 933:175–184.
10. Mao J. Opioid-induced abnormal pain sensitivity: implications in clinical opioid therapy. Pain 2002; 100(3):213–217.
11. Yenari MA, Bell TE, Kotake AN, et al. Dose escalation safety and tolerance study of the competitive NMDA antagonist selfotel (CGS-19755) in neurosurgery patients. Clin Neuropharmacol 1998; 21(1):28–34.
12. Muir KW, Lees KR. Excitatory amino acid antagonists for acute stroke. Cochrane Database Syst Rev 2003; 3:CD001244.
13. Hoyte L, Barber PA, Buchan AM, et al. The rise and fall of NMDA antagonists for ischemic stroke. Curr Mol Med 2004; 4(2):131–136.
14. Wood PL. The NMDA receptor complex: a long and winding road to therapeutics. IDrugs 2005; 8(3):229–235.
15. Parsons CG, Danysz W, Quack G. Memantine is a clinically well tolerated $N$-methyl-D-aspartate (NMDA) receptor antagonist—review of preclinical data. Neuropharmacology 1999; 38:735–767.

16. MacDonald JF, Bartlett MC, Mody I, et al. Actions of ketamine, phencyclidine and MK-801 on NMDA receptor currents in culture mouse hippocampal neurons. J Physiol 1991; 432:483–508.
17. Chizh BA, Cumberbatch MJ, Herrero JF, et al. Stimulus intensity, cell excitation and the *N*-methyl-D-aspartate receptor component of sensory responses in the rat spinal cord in vivo. Neuroscience 1997; 80:251–265.
18. Chizh BA. Low dose ketamine: a therapeutic and research tool to explore *N*-methyl-D-aspartate (NMDA) receptor-mediated plasticity in pain pathways. J Psychopharmacol 2007; 21(3):259–271.
19. Jones MW, McClean M, Parsons CG, et al. The in vivo relevance of the varied channel-blocking properties of uncompetitive NMDA antagonists: test on spinal neurons. Neuropharmacology 2001; 41:50–61.
20. Smith DG, Pekoe GM, Martin LL, et al. The interaction of ketamine with the opiate receptor. Life Sci 1980; 26(10):789–795.
21. Smith DG, Bouchal RL, deSanctis CA, et al. Properties of the interaction between ketamine and opiate binding site in vivo and in vitro. Neuropharmacology 1987; 26:1253–1260.
22. Orser BA, Pennefather PS, MacDonald JF. Multiple mechanisms of ketamine blockade of *N*-methyl-D-aspartate receptors. Anesthesiology 1997; 86(4):903–917.
23. Kapur S, Seeman P. NMDA receptor antagonist ketamine and PCP have direct effects on the dopamine D(2) and serotonin 5-HT(2) receptors—implications for model of schizophrenia. Mol Psychiatry 2002; 7:837–844.
24. Wood PB. A reconsideration of the relevance of systemic low-dose ketamine to the pathophysiology of fibromyalgia. J Pain 2006; 7(9):611–614.
25. Chizh BA, Eide PK. Pain. In: Lodge D, Danysz W, Parsons CG, eds. Therapeutic Potential of Ionotropic Glutamate Receptor Antagonists and Modulators. Johnson City: F.P. Graham publishing Co., 2002:263–300.
26. Chizh BA, Headley PM. NMDA antagonists and neuropathic pain—multiple drug targets and multiple uses. Curr Parm Des 2005; 11:2977–2994.
27. Mikkelsen S, Ilkjaer S, Brennum J, et al. The effect of naloxone on hyperalgesia and ketamine-induced side effects in humans. Anesthesiology 1999; 90:1539–1545.
28. Krystal JH, D'Souza DC. Comment on "ketamine has equal affinity for NMDA receptors and the high-affinity state of the dopamine $D_2$ receptor". Biol Psychiatry 2001; 50:555.
29. Laulin JP, Maurette P, Corcuff JB, et al. The role of ketamine in preventing fentanyl-induced hyperalgesia and subsequent acute morphine tolerance. Anesth Analg 2002; 94(5):1263–1269.
30. Célèrier E, Rivat C, Jun Y, et al. Long-lasting hyperalgesia induced by fentanyl in rats: preventive effect of ketamine. Anesthesiology 2000; 92(2):447–456.
31. Van Elstraete AC, Sitbon P, Trabold F, et al. A single dose of intrathecal morphine in rats induces long-lasting hyperalgesia: the protective effect of prior administration of ketamine. Anesth Analg 2005; 101:1750–1756.
32. Richebe P, Rivat C, Laulin JP, et al. Ketamine improves the management of exaggerated postoperative pain observed in perioperative fentanyl-treated rats. Anesthesiology 2005; 102(2):421–428.
33. Angst MS, Koppert W, Pahl I, at al. Short-term infusion of the mu-opioid agonist remifentanil in humans causes hyperalgesia during withdrawal. Pain 2003; 106:49–57.

34. Joly V, Richebe P, Guignard B, et al. Remifentanil-induced postoperative hyperalgesia and its prevention with small-dose ketamine. Anesthesiology 2005; 103(1):147–155.
35. Singla A, Stojanovic MP, Chen L, et al. A differential diagnosis of hyperalgesia, toxicity, and withdrawal from intrathecal morphine infusion. Anesth Analg 2007; 105(6):1816–1819.
36. Okon T. Ketamine: an introduction for the pain and palliative medicine physician. Pain Physician 2007; 10:493–500.
37. Fine PG. Low-dose ketamine in the management of opioid nonresponsive terminal cancer pain. J Pain Symptom Manage 1999; 17:296–300.
38. Mercadante S, Arcuri E, Tirelli W, et al. Analgesic effect of intravenous ketamine in cancer patients on morphine therapy. J Pain Symptom Manage 2000; 20:246–252.
39. Good P, Tullio F, Jackson K, et al. Prospective audit of short-term concurrent ketamine, opioid and anti-inflammatory "triple-agent" therapy for episodes of acute on chronic pain. Intern Med J 2005; 35:39–44.
40. Jackson K, Ashby M, Martin P, et al. "Burst" ketamine for refractory cancer pain: an open-label audit of 39 patients. J Pain Symptom Manage 2001; 22:834–842.
41. Clements JA, Nimmo WS, Grant IS. Bioavailability, pharmacokinetics, and analgesic activity of ketamine in humans. J Pharm Sci 1982; 71(5):539–542.
42. Fitzgibbon EJ, Hall P, Schroder C, et al. Low dose ketamine as an analgesic adjuvant in difficult pain syndromes: a strategy for conversion from parenteral to oral ketamine. J Pain Symptom Manage 2002; 23:165–170.
43. Kannan TR, Saxena A, Bhatnagar S, et al. Oral ketamine as an adjuvant to oral morphine for neuropathic pain in cancer patients. J Pain Symptom Manage 2002; 23:60–65.
44. Azevedo VM, Lauretti GR, Pereira NL, et al. Transdermal ketamine as an adjuvant for postoperative analgesia after abdominal gynecological surgery using lidocaine epidural blockade. Anesth Analg 2000; 91(6):1479–1482.
45. Jiang JH, Kim DW, Sang NT. Peripheral glutamate receptors contribute to mechanical hyperalgesia in a neuropathic pain model of the rat. Neuroscience 2004; 128:169–176.
46. Christoph T, Reissmuller E, Schiene K, et al. Antiallodynic effects of NMDA glycine B antagonists in neuropathic pain: possible peripheral mechanisms. Brain Res 2005; 1048:218–227.
47. Koppert W, Zeck S, Blunk J, et al. The effects of intradermal fentanyl and ketamine on capsaicin-induced secondary hyperalgesia and flare reaction. Anesth Analg 1999; 89:1521–1527.
48. Gammaitoni A, Gallagher RM, Welz-Bosna M. Topical ketamine gel: possible role in treating neuropathic pain. Pain Med 2000; 1:97–100.
49. Ushida T, Tani T, Kanbara T, et al. Analgesic effects of ketamine ointment in patients with complex regional pain syndrome type 1. Reg Anesth Pain Med 2002; 27:524–528.
50. Lynch ME, Clark AJ, Sawynok J, et al. Topical amitriptyline and ketamine in neuropathic pain syndromes: an open-label study. J Pain 2005; 6(10):644–649.
51. Clerc S, Vuilleumier H, Frascarolo P, et al. Is the effect of inguinal field block with 0.5% bupivacaine on postoperative pain after hernia repair enhanced by addition of ketorolac or S(+) ketamine? Clin J Pain 2005; 21(1):101–105.
52. Ansermino M, Basu R, Vandebeek C, et al. Nonopioid additives to local anesthetics for caudal blockade in children: a systematic review. Paediatr Anaesth 2003; 13(7): 561–573.

53. Subramaniam K, Subramaniam B, Steinbrook RA. Ketamine as adjuvant analgesic to opioids: a quantitative and qualitative systematic review. Anesth Analg 2004; 99(2): 482–495.
54. Chang G, Chen L, Mao J. Opioid tolerance and hyperalgesia. Med Clin North Am 2007; 91(2):199–211.
55. Vielhaber A, Portenoy RK. Advances in cancer pain management. Hematol Oncol Clin North Am 2002; 16(3):527–541.
56. Ossipov MH, Lai J, Vanderah TW, et al. Induction of pain facilitation by sustained opioid exposure: relationship to opioid antinociceptive tolerance. Life Sci 2003; 73:783–800.
57. Fitzgibbon EJ, Viola R. Parenteral ketamine as an analgesic adjuvant for severe pain: development and retrospective audit of a protocol for a palliative care unit. J Palliat Med 2005; 8(1):49–57.
58. Lossignol DA, Obiols-Portis M, Body JJ. Successful use of ketamine for intractable cancer pain. Support Care Cancer 2005; 13(3):188–193.
59. Bell RF, Eccleston C, Kalso E. Ketamine as adjuvant to opioids for cancer pain. A qualitative systematic review. J Pain Symptom Manage 2003; 26:867–875.
60. Fisher K, Coderre TJ, Hagen NA. Targeting the *N*-methyl-D-aspartate receptor for chronic pain management: preclinical animal studies, recent clinical experience and future research directions. J Pain Symptom Manage 2000; 20(5):358–373.
61. Jevtovic-Todorovic V, Wozniak DF, Benshoff ND, et al. A comparative evaluation of neurotoxic properties of ketamine and nitrous oxide. Brain Res 2001; 895:246–247.
62. Stoltz M, Oehen HP, Gerber H. Histological findings after long-term infusion of intrathecal ketamine for chronic pain: a case report. J Pain Symptom Manage 1999; 18:223–228.
63. Fisher K, Hagen NA. Analgesic effect of oral ketamine in chronic neuropathic pain of spinal origin: a case report. J Pain Symptom Manage 1999; 18:61–66.
64. Visser E, Schug SA. The role of ketamine in pain management. Biomed Pharmacother 2006; 60(7):341–348.
65. Elia N, Tramer MR. Ketamine and postoperative pain—a quantitative systematic review of randomized trials. Pain 2005; 113(1–2):61–70.
66. Jevtovic-Todorovic V, Olney JW. Neuroprotective agents. In: Evers AS, Mayes M, eds. Anesthetic pharmacology, physiologic principles and clinical practice. Philadelphia: Churchill Livingstone, 2004:557–572.
67. Farber NB, Kim SH, Dikranian K, et al. Receptor mechanisms and circuitry underlying NMDA antagonist neurotoxicity. Mol Psychiatry 2002; 7:32–43.
68. Prommer E. Ketamine to control pain. J Palliat Med 2003; 6(3):443–446.
69. Kim SH, Price MT, Olney JW, et al. Excessive cerebrocortical release of acetylcholine induced by NMDA antagonists is reduced by GABAergic and $\alpha_2$-adrenergic agonists. Mol Psychiatry 1999; 4:344–352.
70. Handa F, Tanaka M, Nishikawa T, et al. Effects of oral clonidine premedication on side effects of intravenous ketamine anesthesia: a randomized, double-blind placebo-controlled study. J Clin Anesth 2000; 12:19–24.
71. Correll EC, Maleki J, Gracely EJ, et al. Subanesthetic ketamine infusion therapy: a retrospective analysis of a novel therapeutic approach to complex regional pain syndrome. Pain Med 2004; 5(3):263–275.

# 10

# Role of Opioid Rotation and Tapering in Managing Opioid-Induced Hyperalgesia

**Howard S. Smith**

*Department of Anesthesiology, Albany Medical College,*
*Albany, New York, U.S.A.*

## INTRODUCTION

Although gradual escalation of opioid dose in many patients achieves a favorable balance between analgesia and side effects, some patients experience intolerable side effects before adequate analgesia is reached or, alternatively, do not benefit at all. Several strategies can be employed to reduce toxicity, opioid-induced hyperalgesia (OIH), and/or improve analgesia, including more aggressive treatment of side effects, use of coanalgesics or combination opioid analgesics (1), interventional procedures, and use of nonpharmacological interventions. An alternative approach is to change to another opioid in an attempt to allow titration to adequate pain control while limiting side effects (2).

The practice of changing from one opioid to another, referred to as *opioid rotation*, is most commonly undertaken when adequate analgesia is limited by the occurrence of problematic side effects. The principle of rotation is based on the observation that a patient's response can vary from opioid to opioid, for both analgesia and adverse effects. Importantly, an inadequate response or the occurrence of intolerable side effects with one opioid does not necessarily predict a similar response to another (2).

The practical and theoretical advantages of opioid rotation include improved analgesia, reduced side effects and OIH, cost reduction, and improved

*134*

compliance. Disadvantages include problems related to inaccurate conversion tables, limited availability of certain opioid formulations, drug interactions, and the possibility of increased expense. Weighing the advantages and disadvantages is essential prior to making a decision about opioid rotation selection (3). It remains unclear to what extent the manner/technique of rotation, optimal dose/ dose frequency titration, or the choice of different opioids has an impact on clinical outcomes.

## CLINICAL EXPERIENCE

The reported use of opioid rotation varies widely, ranging in frequency from less than 10% to up to 80% of patients (4–7). With the release of a number of new opioids and opioid formulations in recent years, it is likely that the practice has become more frequent. Muller-Busch et al. (8) showed that in some palliative care units, rotation from one long-acting opioid to another occurred less frequently than expected based on the published literature. This suggests that many problems can be managed by adaptation of dosage, route change, or the use of coanalgesics and adjuvants. Furthermore, although there is no robust data to support this, it seems that the practice of opioid rotation is more common in oncology and palliative medicine than in the treatment of patients with persistent noncancer pain.

However, opioid rotation certainly is utilized in the treatment of noncancer pain as well. Grilo et al. (9) studied opioid rotation in 67 patients suffering from low back pain with sciatica in 27 cases, inflammatory arthritis in 14 cases, brachial neuralgia in 6 cases, osteoarthritis in 8 cases, and miscellaneous in 12 cases. The opioid rotations were the substitution of morphine by transdermal fentanyl (9) or by oral hydromorphone in most of the cases. The principal reason for opioid rotation was failure of the first treatment. The mean of VAS improvement was 30 mm ($p < 0.0001$).

Mercadante and Bruera (10) found that opioid rotation results in clinical improvement in at least 50% of patients, with chronic pain presenting with a poor response to a particular opioid; however, a Cochrane review (11) revealed that there are no randomized controls for opioid rotation. The evidence to support the practice is largely anecdotal or based on uncontrolled studies, but switching to a different opioid appears to be a useful maneuver, at least in certain circumstances. The most common aims of opioid rotation are to improve pain control, reduce toxicity, or both. Other indications for opioid rotation include patient convenience, convenience of route, wish for a reduction in invasiveness, and cost (12).

It is probable that actions of glutamate and other excitatory amino acids on *N*-methyl-D-aspartate receptor (NMDA-R) facilitate sensitization of spinal neurons and development of the excitatory symptoms, including OIH (13). Accordingly, administration of NMDA antagonists has been shown to reduce neuroexcitation caused by high-dose morphine (14) and remifentanil in humans

(15), as well as fentanyl (13) and heroin in rodents (16). Consequently, opioids with pure μ-receptor activity may, at least in some patients, induce hyperalgesia (17). In an animal model, the more the fentanyl administered, the more is the sustained hyperalgesia developed (13). Although intuitively, the most direct manner to address the pain of OIH would seemingly be to discontinue or significantly taper the opioid, opioid rotation may also have benefits in certain circumstances.

Okon and George (18) described a case of fentanyl-induced neurotoxicity at 200 μg/hr (e.g., severe allodynia, myoclonus, delirium) and fentanyl-induced hyperalgesia in which all symptoms, including pain/hyperalgesia, resolved with opioid rotation to an opioid for mild to moderate pain.

In addition to cases in which improved analgesia is achieved after switching to a different opioid, opioid rotation may also be useful to alleviate adverse effects from a specific opioid. Wirz et al. (19) conducted a prospective, open-labeled, randomized controlled trial on 100 outpatients with cancer pain and analyzed two separate comparable groups of 50 patients into treatment with hydromorphone (HM) or morphine (M). Mobility, pain, and gastrointestinal symptoms were assessed by the ECOG performance status, selected items of the EORTC questionnaire, and numerical rating scale (NRS). Data were analyzed using descriptive and confirmatory statistics (paired $t$-test, chi-square test, Poisson regression) (19). Demographic and medical data were comparable in both treatment groups. Taking into account different conversion factors, opioid doses [M 94.4 mg/day vs. HM 137.6 (HM/M = 1:5), $p = 0.05$ and HM 206.4 (HM/M = 1:7.5), $p = 0.0002$, respectively] were higher under hydromorphone and NRS of pain (M 2.3 vs. HM 3.6, $p = 0.0002$) lower under morphine (19). It is perceived by some that phenanthrenes with a hydroxyl group in the 6-position (e.g., M) tend to be more emetic than phenanthrenes without a hydroxyl group in the 6-position (e.g., HM). NRS of nausea (M 2.5 vs. HM 1.5; $p = 0.01$), incidences of emesis (M 0.7/day vs. HM 0.1/day, $p = 0.0001$), the consumption of antiemetics (M 26 vs. HM 14, $p = 0.01$), and the number of constipated patients (M 8 vs. HM 2, $p = 0.04$) were higher in the morphine group (19). An extended use of substances for symptom control revealed constipating effects (M 31 vs. HM 13, $p = 0.0003$) and was associated with a higher incidence of constipation in the morphine group/higher laxative use in the morphine group (19).

## POTENTIAL MECHANISMS AND SCIENTIFIC RATIONALE FOR OPIOID ROTATION

The mechanisms behind the success of opioid rotation remain uncertain, and there is little hard evidence that it is, in fact, effective. However, several theories have surfaced to explain why a change to a different opioid may diminish adverse effects and/or improve analgesia. Each opioid may possess different characteristics and/or qualities. Furthermore, there may exist significant variations with respect to various different opioid actions/activities for different opioids, as well as significant variation in responsiveness to different opioids. Although precise mechanisms to entirely explain variation in opioid responsiveness remain uncertain, two potential mechanisms that may help explain some of the variations in opioid responsiveness and variations in adverse effects are differences in opioid metabolism and differences in parmacogenetics (20).

## ADVERSE EFFECTS FROM TOXIC METABOLITES

The accumulation of toxic metabolites may lead to severe side effects in patients on chronic opioid therapy. For example, the primary metabolite of morphine, morphine-6-glucuronide (M6G), is an active compound that is considerably more potent than its parent compound. Morphine-3-glucuronide (M3G) accumulates in patients with renal failure and is a common cause of opioid-related toxicity in such patients (21). The metabolites of other opioids (e.g., dextropropoxyphene and tramadol) also accumulate in renal failure and may contribute to toxicity in the absence of dose reduction. Still other opioids (e.g., fentanyl and alfentanil) are metabolized in the liver to inactivate products and are therefore safer to use in patients with renal failure than morphine. Thus, in a patient with renal impairment, rotating from morphine to an opioid with pharmacodynamics not dependent on renal function should allow for the clearance of toxic metabolites while simultaneously enabling the maintenance or improvement of pain control.

The existing literature has implicated morphine and its toxic metabolites as presumptively contributing to OIH (22–27). Consequently, the existing clinical reports and guidelines suggest opioid rotation, preferentially to agents without known toxic metabolites, such as fentanyl, as one treatment of OIH (28–30). However, as a cautionary vignette, we report a case of neurotoxicity, inclusive of hyperalgesia, in a cancer patient who was associated with treatment with a moderate dose of fentanyl and resolved with discontinuation of the medication.

Neurotoxicity observed with opioid analgesia has frequently been attributed to action of opioid metabolites, such as M3G or hydromorphone-3-glucuronide (24,31). In humans, fentanyl is metabolized to norfentanyl and other similarly inactive metabolites by the *N*-dealkylating cytochrome P450 3A4 isoenzyme. Fentanyl is not known to significantly bind to nonopioid receptors and thereby exert an antiglycinergic effect previously implicated in the development of allodynia, hyperalgesia, and myoclonus (29,32).

## Pharmacogenetics

Considerable evidence is accumulating to suggest genetic variability between individuals and in their ability to metabolize and respond to drugs. For example, codeine is ineffective as an analgesic in about 10% of the Caucasian population due to genetic polymorphisms in the enzyme necessary to O-methylate codeine to morphine, the active metabolite. Other polymorphisms can lead to enhanced metabolism and thus increased sensitivity to codeine's effects (33). Genetic variability in the expression or density of opioid receptors (ORs), receptor affinity, or secondary messenger activation may explain the interindividual variation seen in patients' response to morphine. Similarly, variability in the expression of the enzymes responsible for the metabolism of different opioids may contribute to differences in dose requirements and toxicity. In the future, pharmacogenetic mapping may allow us to predict which opioid will be best suited to a particular individual (34).

The scientific rationale for opioid switching may be appreciated in part by the genetic variation of certain candidate genes that help define an individual patient's unique pharmacokinetics/pharmacodynamics/μ-opioid receptor (MOR) signaling efficiency.

Genetic variation in the multidrug-resistance gene MDR-1 [which encodes for P-glycoprotein, a membrane-bound drug transporter that regulates transfer of opioids across the blood-brain barrier by actively pumping opioids out of the central nervous system (CNS)] may account for the genetic variability in P-glycoprotein activity (35,36). The mutation resulting in the G2677T/A genotype of P-glycoprotein has been demonstrated to alter drug levels (37) and drug-induced side effects (38), though no such studies exist for opioid effects (36).

Investigators have identified more than 100 polymorphisms in the human MOR gene (Oprm), with some variants exhibiting altered binding affinities to different opioids (36,39,40). The best-known polymorphism in the Oprm is the A118G nucleotide substitution, which codes for the amino acid change of asparagine to aspartic acid. It is unclear whether genetic variation in various polymorphisms contributes to variation in the effects of different opioids.


## PHARMACOKINETIC VARIABILITY

### Opioid Metabolizers

Considerable evidence is accumulating to suggest genetic variability between individuals and in their ability to metabolize and respond to drugs. All opioid drugs are substantially metabolized, mainly by the cytochrome P450 system and, to a lesser extent, by UDP-glucuronosyltransferases (UGTs), which are also involved in secondary metabolic pathways. Codeine may be ineffective as an analgesic in about 10% of the Caucasian population due to genetic polymorphisms in the enzyme CYP2D6 necessary to O-methylate codeine to morphine, the active metabolite. Other polymorphisms can lead to enhanced metabolism and thus increased sensitivity to codeine's effects (33). Genetic variability in the expression or density of ORs, receptor affinity, or secondary messenger activation may explain the interindividual variation seen in patients' response to morphine. Similarly, variability in the expression of the enzymes responsible for the metabolism of different opioids may contribute to differences in dose requirements and toxicity. In the future, pharmacogenetic mapping may allow us to predict which opioid will be best suited to a particular individual (34).

Approximately 5% to 10% of Caucasian population in Europe and North America lack the functional action of the CYP2D6 enzyme due to inactive mutations in both alleles of the CYP2D6 gene; they are poor metabolizers (PMs) of debrisoquine and numerous other drugs (41,42). The *CYP2D6* gene is highly polymorphic, with 100 allelic variants identified (43). Of these, *3–*8 are nonfunctional, *9, *10, and *41 have reduced function, and *1, *2, *35, and *41 can be duplicated resulting in greatly increased expression of functional CYP2D6. There are large interethnic differences in the frequencies of these variant alleles (44). The allele frequency of CYP2D6*10 was found to be 52.4% in a Chinese population (45). Patients were categorized into three groups according to the CYP2D6 genotype: patients without CYP2D6*10 (group I, $n = 17$), patients heterozygous for CYP2D6*10 (group II, $n = 26$), and patients homozygous for CYP2D6*10 (group III, $n = 20$) (45). The demographic data among the three groups were comparable. The total consumption of postoperative tramadol for 48 hours in Chinese patients recovering from major abdominal surgery in group III was significantly higher than that in groups I and II (45). Allele combinations determine CYP2D6 phenotype: two nonfunctional alleles $\Rightarrow$ PM status; at least one reduced functional allele $\Rightarrow$ intermediate metabolizer (IM) status; at least one functional allele $\Rightarrow$ extensive metabolizer (EM) status; multiple copies of a functional allele and/or allele with promoter mutation (46) $\Rightarrow$ ultrarapid metabolizer (UM) status. CYP2D6 activity is highly variable in EMs and distributed with differences as much as 10,000-fold among individuals (47). CYP2D6 also catalyzes the conversion of dihydrocodeine, hydrocodone, oxycodone, and tramadol to dihydromorphine, hydromorphone, oxymorphone, and tramadol metabolite M1, respectively (48–51). The metabolic clearance of 10 mg hydrocodone to hydromorphone was eight times faster in EMs ($28 \pm 10.3$ mL/hr kg) than in PMs ($3.4 \pm 2.4$ mL/hr kg). Furthermore, pretreatment with quinidine, a selective CYP2D6 inhibitor, in the EMs reduced their clearance to levels similar to those in PMs ($5.0 \pm 3.6$ mL/hr kg), and the maximal plasma concentration for hydromorphone was five times higher in EMs than in PMs or in EMs pretreated with quinidine (48). Genetic causes may also trigger or modify drug interactions, which in turn can alter the clinical response to opioid therapy. Because of inhibition of CYP2D6, paroxetine increases the steady-state plasma concentrations of (R)-methadone in extensive but not in PMs of debrisoquine/sparteine (52). In addition to CYP2D6, CYP2B6, 2C19, 3A4, and 3A5 isoforms also are involved in opioid metabolism.

The differences in codeine metabolism between EM and PM have been shown to have an impact on patient-controlled analgesia such that a PM received more frequent codeine dosing before leaving the study because of inadequate analgesia compared with the EM group (53). In a study in palliative care patients who were switched from morphine to oxycodone for delirium, the single PM in the group of 12 required the highest dose of oxycodone, had the poorest pain control, and required the greatest number of doses of rescue opioid (54).

In contrast to the enzymes leading to various active or inactive opioid metabolites, other enzymes act to conjugate opioids/opioid metabolites to make them water soluble, thereby facilitating their elimination. UGT2B7 is the predominant enzyme that catalyzes morphine glucuronidation (55), and multiple single nucleotide polymorphisms in the promoter region of UGT2B7 have been reported, which are of unknown significance (56). The UGT 2B7 gene encodes for UGT2B7, the primary hepatic enzyme responsible for glucuronidation of morphine, which results in the formation of two major metabolites: M6G and M3G (55). Functional allelic variants of UGT2B7 may affect hepatic clearance of morphine by altering its enzymatic activity.

Presence of the UDP-glucuronosyltransferase UGT2B7-840G allele is associated with significantly reduced glucuronidation of morphine and thus contributes to the variability in hepatic clearance of morphine in sickle cell disease (57,58).

Campa et al. hypothesized that patients having both good efflux pump functionality (*ABCB1/MDR1* homozygous C/C) and a defective morphine receptor (*OPRM1* homozygous G/G) would be the worst responders to pain relief treatment (59). By contrast, patients with ineffective efflux pump (*ABCB1/MDR1* homozygous T/T) and a functional receptor (*OPRM1* homozygous A/A) were expected to be the best responders (59). Pain relief variability was significantly ($p < 0.0001$) associated with both polymorphisms (59). Combining the extreme genotypes of both genes, the association between patient polymorphism and pain relief improved ($p < 0.00001$), allowing the detection of three groups: strong responders, responders, and nonresponders, with sensitivity close to 100% and specificity more than 70% (59).

## PHARMACODYNAMIC VARIABILITY

### Opioid Receptors

μ-, κ-, and λ-opioid receptors (encoded by the *OPRM1*, *OPRK1*, and *OPRD1* genes, respectively) may all have polymorphisms. Several polymorphic variants of the human *OPRM1* gene have been described (60–63), including variants that alter amino acid sequence of the receptor, as well as properties of receptor function, studied using in vitro expression systems (62,64–66). There is evidence to suggest that MOR mutations may contribute to interindividual variability of the clinical effects of opioids (67).

Splice variants of the MOR (MOR-1A, MOR-1B, MOR-1C, etc.) have been identified, as well as other variants involving alternative splicing at the 3′ or the 5′ end of the mRNA (68). The variants may utilize a different promoter and possess different characteristics/locations/functions. Some variants may respond to morphine but not to M6G and vice versa (68).

Investigators have identified more than 100 polymorphisms in the human MOR gene (Oprm), with some variants exhibiting altered binding affinities to different opioids (36,39,40). The best-known polymorphism in the Oprm is the A118G nucleotide substitution, which codes for the amino acid change of asparagine to aspartic acid.

The single nucelotide polymorphism A118G alters functional properties of the human MOR (69).

Subjects carrying one or two copies of the variant G allele were found to have a reduced response to morphine treatment and a reduced analgesic response to alfentanil (70–72) and M6G (73). Chou et al. (74,75) studied patients who underwent total knee arthroplasty and abdominal total hysterectomy, and they observed that G/G homozygotes have a poorer response to morphine for postoperative pain control than A/A homozygotes or heterozygotes. Klepstad et al. (76) showed that cancer patients homozygous for the G allele required higher doses of morphine to relieve pain.

Lötsch and colleagues investigated the central nervous effects of levomethadone by means of measuring pupil size in a random sample of 51 healthy volunteers for nine hours after oral administration of 0.075 mg/kg levomethadone. Lötsch et al. concluded that among polymorphisms in OPRM1, ABCB1, and CYP genes previously associated with functional consequences in a different context, the most important pharmacogenetic factor modulating the short-term effects of levomethadone is the polymorphism (OPRM1 118A>G) affecting MORs (77).

Ross et al. (2005) compared "opioid switchers" who did not tolerate morphine with "controls" who responded to morphine; their study revealed significant differences in the genotype of the signal transducer and activator of the transcription 6 (STAT-6) gene between "switchers" and "controls." STAT-6 recognition sites may exist in the Oprm gene. STAT-6 may interact with Oprm, altering Oprm expression and affecting different opioid responses (78). Ross et al. found a significant difference in genotype and allelic frequency for the T8622C polymorphism in the β-arrestin-2 gene, which encodes for β-arrestin (an intracellular protein involved in regulating MOR phosphorylation, desensitization, and internalization); this variation is of unclear clinical significance (78).

Polymorphic variations in the catechol-O-methyltransferase (COMT) gene (which encodes for COMT, an enzyme that metabolizes catecholamines and thus may affect CNS neurotransmitters) have been demonstrated to influence μ-opioid neurotransmitter responses to pain stressors (79) and to affect interindividual variation in pain sensitivity (36,80). Furthermore, Rakvag et al. (2005) found a correlation between COMT genotype and morphine dose requirements in cancer patients (81). Other issues that may affect variations in opioid analgesia/actions include drug interactions and incomplete cross-tolerance, as discussed in the following sections.

## Drug Interactions

The metabolism of many opioids is dependent on the cytochrome P450 system. Moreover, many drugs commonly used in palliative care are inducers, inhibitors, or substrates for cytochrome P450 isoforms 3A4 and 2D6 (Table 1). Therefore, comedication with known P450 inhibitors or inducers will affect opioid

**Table 1**  Interaction Between Analgesics, Inducers, and Inhibitors of the Cytochrome
P450 System

| Cytochrome | Substrate | Inhibitor | Inducer |
|---|---|---|---|
| 3A4 | Alfentanil | Fluconazole | Carbamazepine |
| | Fentanyl | Ketoconazole | Phenytoin |
| | | Itraconazole | Erythromycin |
| | | Metronidazole | Omeprazole |
| | | Norfloxacin | |
| Cyclophosphamide | | Fluoxetine | Dexamethasone |
| | | Fluvoxamine | Rifampicin |
| | | Sertraline | Phenobarbital |
| | | Clarithromycin | St. John's wort |
| | | Erythromycin | |
| | | Cannabinoids | |
| 2D6 | Oxycodone | Cimetidine | Phenytoin |
| | Methadone | Paroxetine | Carbamazepine |
| | Morphine | Desipramine | Phenobarbital |
| | Tramadol | Fluoxetine | |
| | Codeine | Haloperidol | |
| | | Sertraline | |
| | | Celecoxib | |

*Source*: From Ref. 2.

metabolism and thus dose requirements and toxicity. Any beneficial or delete-
rious outcome following rotation may reflect changing drug interactions (82).

## Incomplete Cross-tolerance

Incomplete cross-tolerance is a mechanism of action most commonly thought to
explain the perceived benefits of opioid rotation (83–85). Analgesic tolerance is
defined as a state of adaptation in which exposure to a drug induces changes that
result in a diminution of one or more of the drug's effects over time. Incomplete
cross-tolerance has been postulated as the mechanism whereby a patient remains
tolerant to the side effects, but not to the analgesic effect, of an opioid in rotating
from one opioid to another.

 Incomplete cross-tolerance describes patients who are tolerant to high
doses of the first opioid, yet have a lower tolerance to the new opioid. It is a
result of the rate and magnitude of tolerance to side effects being different from
the rate and magnitude of tolerance to pain. Conceivably, a patient will benefit
from a change of opioid only if the cross-tolerance to the analgesic effect is less
than the cross-tolerance to the adverse effects. Postulated mechanisms for
incomplete cross-tolerance include preferential binding to different receptor
subtypes and/or the use of different secondary messenger systems by different

opioids, perhaps related to differences in their chemical structure and receptor binding properties (84).

## SPECIAL CONSIDERATIONS FOR OPIOID ROTATION IN OIH

In patients with OIH, if the clinical situation is amendable to appropriate discontinuation of opioid therapy, this may be the best treatment option. However, if opioid discontinuation does not appear to be in the patient's best interest in the short term, then switching to a different opioid (e.g., opioid rotation) may be the optimal treatment option. Although it may be best to switch to a different class of opioid (e.g., from phenanthrenes to phenylpiperidines), there is no evidence to support algorithms or guidelines in choosing a different opioid for a specific individual patient and each case should be evaluated on an individual basis by experienced pain medicine clinicians/teams.

Some pain medicine experts may advocate that for opioid rotation in the setting of OIH, methadone should be a preferred opioid analgesic. Methadone may be a particularly good agent due to its properties as an NMDA-R antagonist, since the NMDA-R has been implicated as contributing to at least some cases of OIH. Although this strategy may be reasonable, there is no robust evidence to show that methadone is better than other opioids in these circumstances; and there is likely no ideal opioid to switch to for every patient with OIH—each case should be approached individually. More discussion on this particular topic can be found in a separate chapter in this book.

## GENERAL ISSUES OF OPIOID ROTATION

In principle, opioid rotation is an attractive way to achieve a desired benefit, yet many factors (e.g., pharmacokinetics, mixed pain syndromes, opioid side effects, opioid titration, patient preferences) can make this approach difficult. Conversion tables are often inaccurate, opioid choices are limited by formulations and availability, new drug interactions can occur, and there may be increased costs. All of these factors should be considered prior to rotating opioids. Before discarding the current treatment because of adverse side effects or a lack of efficacy, consider readjusting the opioid dose, adding adjuvant analgesics (thus sparing opioids), and utilizing specific treatments for the side effects.

At the same time, through observational studies and clinician experience, opioid rotation is often considered a first-line treatment option when pain control is lacking despite dose increases or when side effects limit titrations. These experiences have been corroborated by experiments in mice showing marked variability in response to morphine (86). Gene splicing has elucidated at least 15 splice variants of the MOR gene (MOR-1), which have variable affinity to different opioids and distinct regional distributions (87). Although studies of specific gene splice variants are not possible in humans, the complexity of the human genome suggests even more interindividual variation.

**Table 2** Key Points for Opioid Rotation

- Utilize an opioid equianalgesic table that is appropriate/relevant for your practice, and use it consistently.
- In deciding on an alternative opioid, consider all patient factors (e.g., What is the best route of drug delivery in this patient? Which drug is most convenient for the patient/ treating team? Is cost going to be an issue? Is the new drug available in the community?).
- In rotating opioids, consider all medical factors that may be relevant (e.g., renal function, liver function, age, comorbidities), and adjust equianalgesic dose based on these factors.
- In rotating to an opioid other than methadone or fentanyl, decrease the equianalgesic dose by 25% to 50%.
- In rotating to methadone, reduce the dose by 75% to 90%.
- In rotating to transdermal fentanyl, maintain the equianalgesic dose.
- In rotating because of uncontrolled pain, consider a lesser dose reduction than usual.
- Ensure that appropriate rescue/breakthrough doses are available. Use 5% to 15% of the total daily opioid dose as a guide, and reassess and retitrate the new opioid.

*Source*: From Ref. 2.

When phenanthrene opioids (morphine, hydromorphone, oxycodone) are used, substitution of the presumed causative agent with an alternative, usually a piperadine derivative (opioid rotation), should be considered as a first-line approach. Clinicians should be cautious when titrating doses for opioid rotation, since acutely switching to significantly higher equivalent doses may lead to adverse effects (including possible respiratory depression), and switching to significantly lower equivalent doses may lead to opioid withdrawal syndrome (88) and/or exacerbation of pain.

Guidelines for opioid rotation have been published based largely on case reports or retrospective analyses of patients with cancer pain (89–91). Although morphine remains the "gold standard" in palliative treatment, there are no rigorous studies providing evidence on the preferred selection of a baseline opioid or on indications for switching to specific alternative opioids. If patients with problems on one opioid are rotated, many symptoms appear to improve regardless of the direction of the switch. The key points that have been widely used for opioid rotation are presented in Table 2.

## DOSE CONVERSION

Conversion doses should be based on an equianalgesic table that provides values for the relative potencies among different opioids (Table 3). However, several limitations of equianalgesic tables must be acknowledged. Most conversion tables are based on studies in which opioid-naive individuals were given single low-dose opioids, without attention to side effects, organ failure, polypharmacy, complications, or the reason for rotation. These studies also failed to take into account the

**Table 3** Equianalgesic Conversion Table

| Name | Equianalgesic dose | | | |
|---|---|---|---|---|
| | Oral | Parenteral | Comments | Precautions and contraindications |
| Morphine | 30 mg | 10 mg | Standard of comparison for opioid analgesics | Clearance of parent drug and active metabolite is prolonged in patients with renal failure |
| Hydromorphone | 4–6 mg | ≈1.5 mg | Exact dose equivalence unclear | |
| Hydrocodone | 20 mg | N/A | 1.5:2 hydrocodone: morphine dose equivalence | Available in the United States combined with acetaminophen; maximum daily dose of acetaminophen is 4 g |
| Oxycodone | 20 mg | ≈5–10 mg[a] | 1.5:2 oxycodone: morphine dose equivalence | Clearance is prolonged in patients with hepatic failure |
| Methadone[b] | 10–20 mg (single dose) (may vary widely) | N/A | Long plasma half-life (24–36 hr), unique characteristics, considerable interindividual difference in pharmacokinetics, cannot be titrated in the same manner as other opioids | Accumulates with repeated dosing, unpredictable pharmacology in individual patients; use with caution |
| Buprenorphine | – | – | Available in three- and seven-day transdermal formulations[c] (see manufacturer's recommendations for morphine dose equivalence range) | – |

*(Continued)*

**Table 3**  Equianalgesic Conversion Table (*Continued*)

| Name | Equianalgesic dose Oral | Parenteral | Comments | Precautions and contraindications |
|------|------|------------|----------|-----------------------------------|
| Oxymorphone[d] | 10 mg | 1 to 1.5 mg[a] | Extended release (ER) matrix slowly releases oxymorphone over 12 hr | – |
| Fentanyl | N/A | 200 μg | Available in transdermal preparation (see manufacturer's recommendations for morphine dose equivalence range) | Considered reasonably safe in patients with renal impairment |

*Source*: Ref. (2).
[a]Parenteral not available in the United States<<end-dots or semi colon>>;
[b]It is extremely important to monitor all patients closely when converting from methadone to other opioid agonists. The ratio between methadone and other opioid agonists may vary widely as a function of previous dose exposure. Methadone has a long half-life and tends to accumulate in the plasma;
[c]Transdermal not available in the United States;
[d]The approximate equivalent doses in this conversion table are only to be used for the conversion from current opioid therapy to oxymorphone extended release (Opana ER). Sum the total daily dose for the opioid and use the approximate equivalent doses to calculate the oxymorphone total equianalgesic daily dose. For patients on a regimen of mixed opioids, calculate the approximate oral oxymorphone dose for each opioid and sum the totals to estimate the total daily equianalgesic oxymorphone dose. The dose of oxymorphone extended release (Opana ER) can be gradually adjusted, preferably at increments of 10 mg every 12 hours every three to seven days, until adequate pain relief and acceptable side effects have been achieved.

interindividual variations that play a prominent role in determining the real conversion for each individual. The variation in published conversion ratios is also a problem. Oxycodone, fentanyl, and methadone show the largest differences among the available conversion tables (92). Small variations in conversion ratios can lead to large differences in calculated equianalgesic doses, especially at higher doses. For example, reported morphine-to-oxycodone ratios have ranged from 1:1 to 2:1.

Methadone deserves special consideration in dose conversion. It has many advantages, including low cost, good oral and rectal absorption, no active metabolites, low tolerance development, and long duration of effect. At the same time, however, its half-life is long and may be unpredictable, with large interindividual variations. This can result in delayed toxicity. Moreover, methadone has been linked to prolongation of the QTc, whereas buprenorphine is associated with less QTc prolongation (93). The conversion dose varies depending on the dose of the original opioid used. At morphine equivalence of less than 90 mg, a conversion of 5:1 (morphine:methadone) is recommended. At morphine equivalence of 90 to 300 mg, a conversion of 6:1 is suggested. For doses of morphine over 300 mg, a rotation of 8:1 is recommended (94). In some individuals, steady-state blood levels are not achieved for four days; therefore, dose adjustments could be considered every four to five days.

Within the last decade, studies and reports of various methadone conversion methodologies have been published (85,95–103) and anecdotal reports of other practice strategies have also appeared in the literature (104). Numerous reviews on the clinical use of methadone discuss the challenges associated with opioid rotation with this drug (94,105–112).

Weschules and Bain performed a systematic review of opioid conversion ratios used with methadone for the treatment of pain (104). They reviewed clinical trials and retrospective analyses, case series, and case reports of human subjects published in the English language between January 1966 and June 2006; review articles and reports with incomplete opioid data were excluded. Twenty-two clinical studies and 19 case reports or series were reviewed ($n = 730$ patients) (104). Methadone rotations were most common in cancer patients ($n = 625$, 88.9%) and those prescribed morphine [$n = 259$ patients, 41.7% of rotations where prerotation opioid was identified ($n = 621$)] or hydromorphone ($n = 234$ patients, 37.7% of rotations). In clinical studies, the most common reason for switching to methadone was a combination of inadequate analgesia and adverse effects ($n = 254$, 38.6%). Despite various approaches, 46% to 89% of rotations were successful. Overall, there was a relatively strong, positive correlation between the previous morphine dose and the final methadone dose and dose ratio, but ratios varied widely (104).

Weschules and Bain (104) concluded that there was no evidence to support the superiority of one method of rotation to methadone over another. Patients may be successfully rotated to methadone despite discrepancies between rotation ratios initially used and those associated with stabilization. Further research is needed to identify patient-level factors that may explain the wide variance in successful methadone rotations (104).

Specifically, lack of reliable equianalgesic conversion ratios to and from methadone increased potency associated with methadone in high doses of another opioid, large interindividual variability in methadone pharmacokinetics, and the potential for numerous drug-drug interactions have made standardized use of methadone difficult (104). Equianalgesic opioid conversion tables, albeit useful for converting most opioid analgesics, have never been shown to contribute to safer, more effective use of methadone in clinical practice.

The conversion methods utilized throughout the review by Weschules and Bain were as follows: oral morphine to parenteral morphine = 3:1 (113,114), parenteral morphine to parenteral hydromorphone = 10:1.5 (113,114), oral morphine to oral hydromorphone = 4:1 (113,114), parenteral morphine to parenteral levorphanol = 5:1 (113,114), and parenteral morphine to parenteral fentanyl = 100:1 (104,113,114). While the equianalgesic opioid conversion tables are less than ideal, most of the ratios provided, with the exception of methadone, are accepted for use in clinical practice (114–117). According to the manufacturer's product insert, the equianalgesic dose of TD fentanyl is provided within a range of OME (118); however, the conversion ratio that is commonly used in clinical practice differs (113,114,119). For the purpose of formulating this review, Weschules and Bain used two conversion strategies for TD fentanyl: (*i*) a straight conversion of oral morphine to TD fentanyl = 100:1 (113,114,120) and (*ii*) a calculated conversion performed by doubling the number of milligrams per hour of TD fentanyl to equal the number of mg of oral morphine/day (113,114,119). In the case of the latter strategy, for example, 50 mg/hr of TD fentanyl was calculated to be 100 mg of OME (104).

Very few studies or cases have described rotations from methadone to another opioid. Four references specifically address this issue ($n = 27$ patients). In a study by Lawlor et al., six such rotations were described (96). A 10:1 (OME: OMeE) dose ratio was used to rotate patients from methadone to morphine; however, unlike the phased approach used for rotating patients from morphine to methadone, the clinicians used an immediate switch (i.e., "stop and go") approach for the reverse rotation (104).

The overall median (range) time to reach stabilization postrotation was four days (4–5 days). There were no significant differences in mean (±SD) pain intensity ratings before and after the switch (72.5±21.8 vs. 55±27.7, respectively; $p= 0.08$) (104). The reported median (lower-upper quartiles) opioid dose ratio for the conversion from methadone to morphine was 8.25:1 (4.37–11.3:1), which was expressed in the direction of morphine to methadone (104).

Mercadante et al. described the outcomes of seven patients rotated from methadone to TD fentanyl using a 1:20 (equivalent to a 5:1 OME:OMeE) conversion ratio (121). The mean prerotation OMeE dose was 30.8 mg/day. The mean [95% confidence interval (CI)] TD fentanyl dose immediately postrotation was 1.54 mg/day (0.49–2.6 mg/day); the mean (95% CI) TD fentanyl dose at the time of stabilization (mean, two days) was 2.20 mg/day (0.46–3.94 mg/day; $p$ value not reported for difference) (121). Treatment was considered successful in all seven patients, as demonstrated by improvements in mean (95% CI) pain [5.8 (4.1–7.6) vs. 2.6 (1.5–3.6); $p < 0.05$] and distress scores [10.7 (7.4–14.0) vs. 6.1 (3.1–9.1); $p < 0.05$] at stabilization compared with baseline. Because the TD fentanyl doses at the time of stabilization were 30% higher than initially calculated, the clinicians suggested that a 1:13 (as opposed to 1:20) ratio may have been more accurate for the conversion (121). On the basis of the conversion to an OME:OMeE ratio outlined in the review by Weschules and Bain, the ratios associated with the initial TD fentanyl and prerotation OMeE dose would be approximately 4.2 to 5:1 and 6 to 7:1, depending on the TD fentanyl to OME conversion method used (104).

It may be less important to determine an exact opioid ratio when performing a methadone conversion than it is to assure that the patient is an appropriate candidate for methadone rotation, the switch is carried out over a time period consistent with the therapeutic goals, and the patient is monitored closely by medical staff throughout the process (104). With the right patient environment and circumstances, opioid rotation to methadone can be done at home (122).

Two different modalities, generally known as *slow switching* and *rapid switching*, have been proposed for this opioid substitution (121). In the slow switching modality, the Edmonton model (123) and the Milan model (102), morphine is decreased gradually by thirds on three successive days and is replaced by methadone at variable dose ratios (e.g., from 4:1 to 12:1) (121). In the rapid switching modality, the U.K. model (124) and the Palermo model (85), previously administered morphine is stopped and replaced by methadone. In the U.K. model, a daily methadone dose of 10% of the morphine dose (with a maximum of 30 mg) is given for six days. On day 6, the amount of methadone taken over the past two days is converted into an every-12-hour regime (121).

Benitez-Rosario et al. evaluated a protocol for switching opioid from transdermal fentanyl to oral methadone in 17 patients with cancer (121). Reasons for switching were uncontrolled pain (41.1% of patients) and neurotoxic side effects (58.9% of patients). After transdermal fentanyl withdrawal, the scheduled daily methadone doses (administered every 8 hours) were administered 8 to 12, 12 to 16, 16 to 18 hours, or 18 to 24 hours afterward, depending on whether previous transdermal fentanyl doses were $\leq 100$ µg/hr, 100 to 200 µg/hr, 200 to 300 µg/hr, or >300 µg/hr, respectively (121). The starting methadone dose was calculated according to a two-step conversion between transdermal fentanyl:oral morphine (1:100 ratio) and oral morphine:oral methadone (5:1 ratio or 10:1 ratio) (121).

Opioid rotation was fully or partially effective in 80% and 20%, respectively, of patients with somatic pain (121). Neuropathic pain was not affected by opioid switching. Delirium and myoclonus were completely eliminated in 80% and 100% of patients, respectively, after opioid switching (121). A positive linear correlation was obtained between the fentanyl and methadone doses (Pearson $r$, 0.851). Previous fentanyl doses were not correlated with the final fentanyl:methadone dose ratios (Spearman's $r$, $-0.327$).

Benitez-Rosario et al. concluded that the protocol studied provided a safe approach for switching from transdermal fentanyl to oral methadone, improving the balance between analgesia and side effects in patients with cancer (121).

Morita et al. investigated the efficacy of opioid rotation from morphine to fentanyl in symptom palliation of morphine-induced delirium. Twenty cancer patients with morphine-induced delirium underwent opioid rotation to fentanyl; morphine was substituted with transdermal fentanyl in 9 patients and parenteral fentanyl in 11 patients. Total opioid dose increased from 64 mg oral morphine equivalent/day (day 0) to 98 mg/day (day 7), and the median increase in total opioid dose was 42%. Treatment success, defined as the Memorial Delirium Assessment Scale (MDAS) score below 10 and pain score of 2 or less, was obtained in 13 patients on day 3 and 18 patients on day 7. The mean MDAS score significantly decreased from 14 (day 0) to 6.4 and 3.6 (Days 3 and 7, respectively,

$p < 0.001$). Pain scores significantly decreased from 2.2 (day 0) to 1.3 and 1.1 on the categorical verbal scale (days 3 and 7, respectively, $p < 0.001$); from 2.6 (day 0) to 1.6 and 1.3 on the Schedule for Team Assessment Scale (STAS) (days 3 and 7, respectively, $p < 0.001$). Symptom scores of dry mouth, nausea, and vomiting significantly decreased, and performance status significantly improved. Morita et al. (125) concluded that opioid rotation from morphine to fentanyl may be effective in alleviating delirium and pain in cancer patients with morphine-induced delirium. Although no well-designed, large-scale prospective studies have attempted to compare commonly used opioids with one another with respect to constipating effects, codeine appears to be associated with a relatively high incidence of constipation. Staats et al. (126) retrospectively studied 1836 patients receiving treatment with transdermal fentanyl, sustained-released oxycodone, and sustained-release morphine. Patients receiving transdermal fentanyl had a lower risk of developing constipation than those taking either of the other two strong opioids. The claim of a lower incidence of constipation with transdermal fentanyl is supported by other studies (127,128).

Tarcatu et al. describe a case of severe opioid-induced pruritus following systemic morphine administration (129). Symptoms did not resolve after administration of antihistamines or rotation to fentanyl or hydromorphone, but oral oxycodone and very low-dose intravenous naloxone did alleviate the patient's itching (129).

Mercadante et al. (130) assessed plasma changes of fentanyl and methadone underlying the clinical events occurring during opioid switching (130). Eighteen patients with cancer, receiving transdermal fentanyl with uncontrolled pain and/or moderate to severe opioid adverse effects, were switched to oral methadone using an initial fixed ratio of 1:20. Fentanyl patches were removed and the first of three daily doses of methadone was started concurrently. Blood samples were obtained at intervals after removing the fentanyl patch and at five-hour intervals for the first 25 hours (130). Methadone plasma concentration increased from 2 to 245 ng/mL, after 25 hours (130). A successful switch (considered a decrease in the pain intensity and distress care) was determined the day after in seven patients, while four patients did not respond favorably (effective switching, 63%). No differences in plasma concentration pattern of the two opioids were found between patients considered responders and non-responders (130). Despite the many advantages of methadone, the variable conversion ratios and its unpredictable half-life make this a difficult medication to use unless the provider is experienced with it.

Once the equianalgesic dose of the new opioid has been calculated, the dose should be adjusted because of incomplete cross-tolerance. When switching, it is prudent to decrease the equianalgesic dose by 25% to 50%—with two exceptions. First, if the new opioid is methadone, the dose should be reduced by 75% to 90%. Second, if the new opioid is transdermal fentanyl, the equianalgesic dose should not be reduced. The dose should be further adjusted based on medical conditions and pain characteristics.

Wirz et al. (131) prospectively studied the technique of opioid rotation to oral sustained-release hydromorphone for controlling pain and symptoms in out-patients with cancer pain. Rotation was successful in 64% of patients experiencing pain (60%), and gastrointestinal (32%) and central (26%) symptoms under oral morphine (38%), transdermal dentanyl (22%), tramadol (20%), oxycodone (12%), or sublingual buprenorphine (8%) (131). NRS of pain (4.1 to 3.2; $p = 0.015$), gastrointestinal symptoms, especially defecation rates ($p = 0.04$), and incidence of insomnia improved after an increase in morphine-equivalent doses from 108.9 to 137.6 mg/day, without modifying concomitant analgesics or coanalgesics (131).

Akiyama et al. (132) retrospectively evaluated the analgesic effects and adverse effects of fentanyl patch among 22 cancer patients (11 men and 11 women) who were switched from morphine to a transdermal fentanyl patch. There were wide variations of conversion ratio with a mean of 96.6 (132).

Narabayashi et al. (133) prospectively investigated the efficacy of opioid rotation from oral morphine to oral oxycodone in 25 cancer patients who had difficulty in continuing oral morphine treatment because of inadequate analgesia and/or intolerable side effects. In spite of intense pain, the morphine daily dose could not be increased in most patients before the study because of intolerable side effects. However, switching to oral oxycodone allowed approximately 1.7-fold increase as morphine equivalent dose. Consequently, 84.0% (21/25) of patients achieved adequate pain control (133). By the end of the study, all patients except one had tolerated the morphine-induced intolerable side effects (i.e., nausea, vomiting, constipation, drowsiness) by switching to oxycodone irrespective of renal function (133).

## SUPPLEMENTAL MEDICATION DURING CONVERSION

Because it is difficult to predict a patient's response to a new opioid, care should always be taken to achieve analgesia without excessive dosing. Especially as incomplete cross-tolerance is unpredictable, rotating to a percentage of the equianalgesic dose is prudent. This may, in turn, result in "underdosing," resulting in increased pain; therefore, short-acting breakthrough medication must be made available. After the steady state of the new opioid is achieved and the usage of the breakthrough medication is known, increases in the new opioid can be appropriately calculated.

## CHANGE OF ROUTE

In addition to a change of drug, opioid rotation may also involve a change in route of drug delivery (e.g., a rotation from oral morphine to rectal morphine or subcutaneous fentanyl). Some believe that a change of route rather than a change of opioid is the most logical means of instigating an opioid rotation (134); the issue is whether changing the route allows for a dose increase and effective analgesia without an increase in side effects. This may hold true for those drugs with active metabolites that undergo extensive first-pass metabolism when given orally. Kalso et al. (135) published a small, double-blind crossover study in which patients were randomized to receive epidural and subcutaneous morphine. There was no difference in effectiveness or acceptability between arms, and both treatments provided better pain relief with fewer adverse effects compared to the prestudy oral morphine treatment. Enting et al. (2002) evaluated the efficacy of parenteral opioids (morphine, fentanyl, and sufentanil) in 100 patients who had failed conventional opioids (codeine, tramadol, morphine, methadone, and transdermal fentanyl). The authors reported an improved balance between analgesia and side effects in 71% of the patients. Furthermore, there was no difference between the patients who changed opioid and route and those who changed route alone (136).

## KEY POINTS FOR OPIOID ROTATION

- Utilize an opioid equianalgesic table that is appropriate/relevant for your practice, and use it consistently.
- In deciding on an alternative opioid, consider all patient factors (e.g., What is the best route of drug delivery in this patient? Which drug is most convenient for the patient/treating team? Is cost going to be an issue? Is the new drug available in the community?).
- In rotating opioids, consider all medical factors that may be relevant (e.g., renal function, liver function, age, comorbidities) and adjust equianalgesic dose based on these factors.
- In rotating to an opioid other than methadone or fentanyl, decrease the equianalgesic dose by 25% to 50%.
- In rotating to methadone, reduce the dose by 75% to 90%.
- In rotating to transdermal fentanyl, maintain the equianalgesic dose.
- In rotating because of uncontrolled pain, consider a lesser dose reduction than usual.
- Ensure that appropriate rescue/breakthrough doses are available. Use 5% to 15% of the total daily opioid dose as a guide, and reassess and retitrate the new opioid.

Although the above-mentioned recommendations encourage the utilization of an opioid equianalgesic conversion table, health-care providers must keep in mind that there is significant variability among opioids and significant differences among patients. Clinicians need to "practice medicine" and "actively decide" the most appropriate opioid dose to start with, tailoring their decisions to specific individual patients, rather than simply "robotically" calculating an opioid dose and prescribing this amount without deciding whether any adjustments are needed. Subsequent close patient follow-up and careful opioid titration should ensue in attempts to achieve optimal analgesia with minimal adverse effects (2).

## OPIOID TAPERING

In situations that require discontinuation of opioid therapy or a significant dose reduction in opioid therapy, a gradual opioid taper intuitively seems the best approach; however, few literature sources discuss opioid tapering. In general, the time needed for smooth opioid tapering with very high pretaper opioid doses that patients have been taking for many years may be significantly longer than this. General taper guidelines include reducing the opioid by 10% daily for 10 days or 5% daily for 20 days (137); reducing by 25% to 50% every 6 to 8 hours for opioids given for less than one week and a 20% initial reduction for opioids given for over a week with subsequent reductions of 10% every 12 hours (138); and reducing 25% of the dose in four divided doses with subsequent reductions of 50% every two days (139,140). The American Pain Society (1999) recommended tapering 50% of the previous daily dose at six-hour intervals for two days, then reducing by 25% every two days until reaching a total dose of 30 mg a day of oral morphine in adults or 0.6 mg/kg a day in children. After two days at the minimum dose, the opioid is discontinued (140).

Gradually tapering the pretaper opioid dose over 5 to 10 days may be the most convenient strategy (141). A successful taper of low to moderate doses of opioids administered for fewer than five days can be accomplished within three to four days, but the time required for tapering increases proportionately if the opioid has been given for greater than five days (140,142). Parran and Pederson evaluated the use of an opioid taper guideline in a research study and found that the use of an opioid taper algorithm appeared to improve the tapering practice for nursing without adversely affecting patient care (140). For patients who had been on opioids less than one week prior to tapering, the algorithm directed nurses to taper the pretaper opioid dose by 10% every eight hours (140). For patients on opioids one week or longer, nurses were directed to taper the pretaper opioid dose by 10% every 12 hours. Thus, unadjusted opioid tapering every eight hours would result in completed tapers in 3.33 days, and tapers decreased every 12 hours would be completed in five days (140).

## OPIOID WITHDRAWAL SYNDROME

All opioids lead to (given long enough in high enough doses) physical dependence with a concomitant withdrawal syndrome upon abrupt cessation of opioid therapy. In addition to abrupt opioid cessation, opioid withdrawal syndrome (OWS) can be precipitated in patients on opioid therapy by administrating an opioid antagonist, an opioid agonist-antagonist (e.g., butorphanol), tapering the opioid dose too quickly, or switching to certain short-acting opioids (88) (especially if they are not dosed with adequate frequency). The severity/duration/onset of the OWS may vary considerably between different individuals and may also vary due to the opioid dose, route of administration, and specific opioid agent (e.g., the onset of OWS after cessation of opioid therapy from a longer-acting opioid agent such as methadone is somewhat delayed as compared with morphine). The OWS may consist of nausea, vomiting, diarrhea, insomnia, yawning, rhinorrhea, piloerection, perspiration (sweating), lacrimation, tremor, mydriasis, hot and cold flashes, restlessness, muscle twitches/myoclonus, abdominal cramps, and anxiety. Furthermore, opioid withdrawal hyperalgesia (OWH) may occur with OWS; and in a patient treated with a short-acting opioid at an inadequate frequency, it may have to be distinguished from OIH (143).

The most commonly used tool in the United States is the clinical opiate withdrawal scale (COWS), which is one clinician-administered instrument that rates 11 common opiate withdrawal signs or symptoms, with each rated from zero to four or five (144). The maximum achievable score is 48.

The degree of clinical opiate withdrawal corresponds to the sum of all 11 items in the following manner: 5 to 12 is mild withdrawal; 13 to 24 moderate; 25 to 36 moderately severe; and greater than 36 severe withdrawal. The Adjective Rating Scale for Withdrawal (ARSW) (145) is a 16-item assessment of symptoms of withdrawal rated from 0 (none) to 9 (severe) by the study subject, and is based on his or her subjective withdrawal discomfort.

The modified version of the Objective Opioid Withdrawal Scale (OOWS) rates 13 observable symptoms of withdrawal (including yawning, rhinnorhea, piloerection, perspiration. Lacrimation, tremor, mydriasis, hot and cold flashes, restlessness, muscle twitches, abdominal cramps, and anxiety)—on a 4-point scale (0: not present, 1: mild, 2: moderate, 3: severe) (146). Gossop developed a 10-item short opiate withdrawal scale (SOWS) in 1990 (147).

One treatment for opioid withdrawal syndrome (OWS) is to administer opioids, however not uncommonly; clinicians may be trying to avoid this. Maintenance therapy with methadone or buprenorphine may be another option [opioid substitution therapy appears to achieve similar benefits across a wide range of countries (148)]; however, clinicians may be aiming for opioid cessation. Although certain investigators have proposed nalbuphine (149) or tramadol (150) in efforts to attenuate OWS, I do not feel these are optimal agents for this purpose.

## AMELIORATION OF OWS

The best-studied agents to ameliorate OWS are α-2 adrenergic agonists (e.g., clonidine, lofexidine) (151,152). Other agents that may be somewhat useful for amelioration of OWS include venlafaxine (153), gabapentin (154), topiramate (155), carbamazepine/mianserin (156), and baclofen (157). Clearly, more research needs to be done. In the future, there may be utility for Chinese herbal medicine in efforts to attenuate OWS (158). Additionally, potential future agents may include corticotrophin-releasing factor (CRF) 1 receptor antagonists (159), selective melanocortin 4 receptor antagonists (160), or selective nuclear factor—κB inhibitors (161).

## SUMMARY

Opioid rotation is a potentially useful strategy, which may be utilized when clinicians are faced with inadequate analgesia, OIH, and/or intolerable opioid-induced adverse effects with existing opioid therapy. Opioid rotation is just one of multiple different strategies to approach these situations. A good working knowledge base of practical opioid pharmacology and opioid treatment options combined with the judgment of experienced pain clinicians may lead to optimal decision making in patient care. Further research is needed in this area, as optimal opioid rotation choices in various situations remain unclear.

## REFERENCES

1. Smith HS. Combination opioid analgesics. Pain Physician 2008; 11(2):201–214.
2. McCarberg BH, Smith HS. Optimizing pharmacologic outcomes: principles of opioid rotation. In: Smith HS, ed. Opioid Therapy in the 21st Century. New York, NY: Oxford University Press, 2008:59–70.
3. Estfan B, LeGrand SB, Walsh D, et al. Opioid rotation in cancer patients: pros and cons. Oncology 2005; 19(4):511–516.
4. Cherny NJ, Chang V, Frager G, et al. Opioid pharmacotherapy in the management of cancer pain. Cancer 1995; 76:1283–1293.
5. Hawley P, Forbes K, Hanks GW. Opioids, confusion and opioid rotation. Palliat Med 1998; 12:63–64.
6. Fainsinger R. Opioids, confusion and opioid rotation. Palliat Med 1998; 12:463–464.
7. Kloke M, Rapp M, Bosse B, et al. Toxicity and/or insufficient analgesia by opioid therapy: risk factors and the impact of changing the opioid. A retrospective analysis of 273 patients observed at a single center. Support Care Cancer 2000; 8:479–486.
8. Muller-Busch HC, Lindena G, Tietz K, et al. Opioid switch in palliative care, opioid choice by clinical need and opioid availability. Eur J Pain 2005; 9(5):571–579.
9. Grilo RM, Bertin P, Scotto di Fazano C, et al. Opioid rotation in the treatment of joint pain. A review of 67 cases. Joint Bone Spine 2002; 69(5):491–494.
10. Mercadante S, Bruera E. Opioid switching: a systematic and critical review. Cancer Treat Rev 2006; 32:304–315.
11. Quigley C. Opioid switching to improve pain relief and drug tolerability. Cochrane Database Syst Rev 2004; 3:CD004847.
12. Cherny N, Ripamonti C, Pereira J, et al., Expert Working Group of the European Association of Palliative Care Network. Strategies to manage the adverse effects of oral morphine: an evidence-based report. J Clin Oncol 2001; 19(9):2542–2554.
13. Célèrier E, Rivat C, Jun Y, et al. Long-lasting hyperalgesia induced by fentanyl in rats: preventive effect of ketamine. Anesthesiology 2000; 92(2):465–472.
14. Lufty K, Woodward RM, Keana JF, Weber E. Inhibition of clonic seizure-like excitatory effects induced by intrathecal morphine using two NMDA receptor antagonists: MK-801 and ACEA-1011. Eur J Pharmacol 1994; 252(3):261–266.
15. Angst MS, Koppert W, Pahl I, et al. Short-term infusion of the mu-opioid agonist remifentanil in humans causes hyperalgesia during withdrawal. Pain 2003; 106 (1e2):49–57.

16. Célèrier E, Laulin JP, Corcuff JB, et al. Progressive enhancement of delayed hyperalgesia induced by repeated heroin administration: a sensitization process. J Neurosci 2001; 21(11):4074–4080.
17. Guignard B, Bossard AE, Coste C, et al. Acute opioid tolerance: intraoperative remifentanil increases postoperative pain and morphine requirement. Anesthesiology 2000; 93(2):409–417.
18. Okon TR, George ML. Fentanyl-induced neurotoxicity and paradoxic pain. J Pain Symptom Manage. 2008; 35(3):327–333.
19. Wirz S, Wartenberg HC, Nadstawek J. Less nausea, emesis, and constipation comparing hydromorphone and morphine? A prospective open-labeled investigation on cancer pain. Support Care Cancer 2008; 16(9):999–1009.
20. Smith HS. Variations in opioid responsiveness. Pain Physician 2008; 11(2):237–248.
21. Osborne R, Joel S, Slevin M. Morphine intoxication in renal failure: the role of morphine-6-glucuronide. Br Med J 1986; 292:1548–1549.
22. Smith MT, Watt JA, Cramond T. Morphine-3-glucuronide potent antagonist of morphine analgesia. Life Sci 1990; 47(6):579–585.
23. De Conno F, Caraceni A, Martini C, et al. Hyperalgesia and myoclonus with intrathecal infusion of high-dose morphine. Pain 1991; 47(3):337–339.
24. Rozan JP, Kahn CH, Warfield CA. Epidural and intravenous opioid-induced neuroexcitation. Anesthesiology 1995; 83(4):860–863.
25. Kronenberg MF, Laimer I, Rifici C, et al. Epileptic seizure associated with intracerebroventricular and intrathecal morphine bolus. Pain 1998; 75(2–3):383–387.
26. Sjögren P, Thunedborg LP, Christrup L, et al. Is development of hyperalgesia, allodynia and myoclonus related to morphine metabolism during long-term administration? Six case histories. Acta Anaesthesiol Scand 1998; 42(9):1070–1075.
27. Andersen G, Christrup LL, Sjøgren P. Morphine metabolism-pharmacokinetics and pharmacodymics. Ugeskr Laeger 1997; 159(22):3383–3386.
28. Sjögren P, Jensen NH, Jensen TS. Disappearance of morphine-induced hyperalgesia after discontinuing or substituting morphine with other opioid agonists. Pain 1994; 59(2):313–316.
29. Hagen N, Swanson R. Strychnine-like multifocal myoclonus and seizures in extremely high-dose opioid administration: treatment strategies. J Pain Symptom Manage 1997; 14(1):51–58.
30. Mercadante S, Arcuri E. Hyperalgesia and opioid switching. Am J Hosp Palliat Care 2005; 22(4):291–294.
31. Andersen G, Christrup L, Sjögren P. Relationships among morphine metabolism, pain and side effects during long-term treatment: an update. J Pain Symptom Manage 2003; 25(1):74–91.
32. Bartlett SE, Dodd PR, Smith MT. Pharmacology of morphine and morphine-3-glucuronide at opioid, excitatory amino acid, GABA and glycine binding sites. Pharmacol Toxicol 1994; 75(2):73–81.
33. Eichelbaum M, Evert B. Influence of pharmacogenetics on drug disposition and response. Clin Exp Pharmacol Physiol 1996; 23:983–985.
34. Roses A. Pharmacogenetics and future drug development and delivery. Lancet 2000; 355:1358–1361.
35. Marzolini C, Paus E, Buclin T, et al. Polymorphisms in human MDR1 (P-glycoprotein): recent advances and clinical relevance. Clin Pharmacol Ther 2004; 75:13–33.

36. Ross JR, Riley J, Quigley C, et al. Clinical pharmacology and pharmacotherapy of opioid switching in cancer patients. Oncologist 2006; 11:765–773.
37. Kim RB, Leake BF, Choo EF, et al. Identification of functionally variant MDR1 alleles among European Americans and Africans Americans. Clin Pharmacol Ther 2001; 70:189–199.
38. Yamauchi A, Ieiri I, Kataoka Y, et al. Neurotoxicity induced by tacrolimus after liver transplantation: relation to genetic polymorphisms of the ABCBI (MDR1) gene. Transplantation 2002; 74:571–572.
39. Surratt CK, Johnson PS, Moriwaki A, et al. Mu opiate receptor. Charged transmembrane domain amino acids are critical for agonist recognition and intrinsic activity. J Biol Chem 1994; 269:20548–20533.
40. Pil J, Tytgat J. The role of the hydrophilic Asn230 residue of the mu-opioid receptor in the potency of various opioid agonists. Br J Pharamacol 2001; 134:496–506.
41. Sachse C, Brockmoller J, Bauer S, Roots I. Cytochrome P450 2D6 variants in a Caucasian population: allele frequencies and phenotypic consequences. Am J Hum Genet 1997; 60:284–295.
42. Eckhardt K, Li S, Ammon S, et al. Same incidence of adverse drug events after codeine administration irrespective of the genetically determined differences in morphine formation. Pain 1998; 76:27–33.
43. Sim S, Ingelman-Sundberg M, Daly AK, Nebert DW. Home page of the Human Cytochrome P450 (CYP) Allele Nomenclature, 2006. Available at: http://www.cypalleles.ki.se/.
44. Zanger UM, Raimundo S, Eichelbaum M. Cytochrome P450 2D6: overview and update on pharmacology, genetics, biochemistry. Naunyn-Schmiedeberg's Arch Pharmacol 2004; 369:23–37.
45. Wang G, Zhang H, He F, Fang X. Effect of the CYP2D6*10 C188T polymorphism on postoperative tramadol analgesia in a Chinese population. Eur J Clin Pharmacol 2006; 62:927–931.
46. Løvlie R, Daly AK, Matre GE, et al. Polymorphisms in CYP2D6 duplication-negative individuals with the ultrarapid metabolizer phenotype: a role for the CYP2D6*35 allele in ultrarapid metabolism? Pharmacogenetics 2001; 11:45–55.
47. Bertilsson L, Dahl ML, Ekqvist B, et al. Genetic regulation of the disposition of psychotropic drugs. In: Meltzer HY, Nerozzi D, eds. Current Practices and Future Developments in the Pharmacotherapy of Mental Disorders. Amsterdam: Elsevier, 1991:73–80.
48. Otton SV, Schadel M, Cheung SW, et al. CYP2D6 phenotype determines the metabolic conversion of hydrocodone to hydromorphone. Clin Pharmacol Ther 1993; 54:463–472.
49. Kirkwood LC, Nation RL, Somogyi AA. Characterization of the human cytochrome P450 enzymes involved in the metabolism of dihydrocodeine. Br J Clin Pharmacol 1997; 44:549–555.
50. Subrahmanyam V, Renwick AB, Walters DG, et al. Identification of cytochrome P-450 isoforms responsible for *cis*-tramadol metabolism in human liver microsomes. Drug Metab Dispos 2001; 29:1146–1155.
51. Lalovic B, Phillips B, Risler LL, et al. Quantitative contribution of CYP2D6 and CYP3A to oxycodone metabolism in human liver and intestinal microsomes. Drug Metab Dispos 2004; 32:447–454.

52. Lötsch J, Skarke C, Liefhold J, et al. Genetic predictors of the clinical response to opioid analgesics: clinical utility and future perspectives. Clin Pharmacokinet 2004; 43:983–1013.

53. Persson K, Sjöström S, Sigurdardottir I, et al. Patient-controlled analgesia (PCA) with codeine for postoperative pain relief in ten extensive metabolisers and one poor metaboliser of dextromethorphan. Br J Clin Pharmacol 1995; 39:182–186.

54. Maddocks I, Somogyi A, Abbott F, et al. Attenuation of morphine-induced delirium in palliative care by substitution with infusion of oxycodone. J Pain Symptom Manage 1996; 12:182–189.

55. Coffman BL, Rios GR, King CD, et al. Human UGT2B7 catalyzes morphine glucuronidation. Drug Metab Dispos 1997; 25:1–4.

56. Duguay Y, Báár C, Skorpen F, et al. A novel functional polymorphism in the uridine diphosphate-glucuronosyltransferase 2B7 promoter with significant impact on promoter activity. Clin Pharmacol Ther 2004; 75:223–233.

57. Darbari DS, Minniti CP, Rana S, et al. Pharmacogenetics of morphine: potential implications in sickle cell disease. Am J Hematol 2008; 83(3):233–236.

58. Darbari DS, van Schaik RH, Capparelli EV, et al. UGT2B7 promoter variant −840G>A contributes to the variability in hepatic clearance of morphine in patients with sickle cell disease. Am J Hematol 2008; 83(3):200–202.

59. Campa D, Gioia A, Tomei A, et al. Association of ABCB1/MDR1 and OPRM1 gene polymorphisms with morphine pain relief. Clin Pharm Ther 2008; 83(4):559–566.

60. Bergen AW, Kokoszka J, Peterson R, et al. Mu opioid receptor gene variants: lack of association with alcohol dependence. Mol Psychiatry 1997; 2:490–494.

61. Berrettini WH, Hoehe MR, Ferraro TN, et al. Human mu opioid receptor gene polymorphisms and vulnerability to substance abuse. Addict Biol 1997; 2:303–308.

62. Bond C, LaForge KS, Tian M, et al. Single nucleotide polymorphism in the human mu opioid receptor gene alters beta-endorphin binding and activity: possible implications for opiate addiction. Proc Natl Acad Sci U S A 1998; 95:9608–9613.

63. Hoehe MR, Kopke K, Wendel B, et al. Sequence variability and candidate gene analysis in complex disease: association of mu opioid receptor gene variation with substance dependence. Hum Mol Genet 2000; 9:2895–2908.

64. Koch T, Kroslak T, Averbeck M, et al. Allelic variation S268P of the human mu-opioid receptor affects both desensitization and G protein coupling. Mol Pharmacol 2000; 58:328–334.

65. Befort K, Filliol D, Decaillot FM, et al. A single nucleotide polymorphic mutation in the human mu-opioid receptor severely impairs receptor signaling. J Biol Chem 2001; 276:3130–3137.

66. Margas W, Zubkoff I, Schuler HG, et al. Modulation of $Ca^{2+}$ channels by heterologously expressed wild-type and mutant human μ-opioid receptors (hMOR) containing the A118G single nucleotide polymorphism. J Neurophysiol 2007; 97: 1058–1067.

67. Lötsch J, Geisslinger G. Are mu-opioid receptor polymorphisms important for clinical opioid therapy? Trends Mol Med 2005; 11:82–89.

68. Pasternak GW. Molecular biology of opioid analgesia. J Pain Symptom Manage 2005; 29:2–9.

69. Korslak T, LaForge KS, Gianotte RJ, et al. The single nucelotide polymorphism A118G alters functional properties of the human mu opioid receptor. J Neurochem 2007; 103:77–87.

70. Romberg RR, Olofsen E, Bijl H, et al. Polymorphism of mu-opioid receptor gene (OPRM1:c.118A>G) does not protect against opioid-induced respiratory depression despite reduced analgesic response. Anesthesiology 2005; 102:522–530.

71. Oertel BG, Schmidt R, Schneider A, et al. The mu-opioid receptor gene polymorphism 118A>G depletes alfentanil-induced analgesia and protects against respiratory depression in homozygous carriers. Pharmacogenet Genomics 2006; 16: 625–636.

72. Lötsch J, Geisslinger G. Relevance of frequent [mu]-opioid receptor polymorphisms for opioid activity in healthy volunteers. Pharmacogenomics J 2006; 6:200–210.

73. Skarke C, Darimont J, Schmidt H, et al. Analgesic effects of morphine and morphine-6-glucuronide in a transcutaneous electrical pain model in healthy volunteers. Clin Pharmacol Ther 2003; 73:107–121.

74. Chou WY, Yang LC, Lu HF, et al. Association of mu-opioid receptor gene polymorphism (A118G) with variations in morphine consumption for analgesia after total knee arthroplasty. Acta Anaesthesiol Scand 2006; 50:787–792.

75. Chou WY, Wang CH, Liu PH, et al. Human opioid receptor A118G polymorphism affects intravenous patient-controlled analgesia morphine consumption after total abdominal hysterectomy. Anesthesiology 2006; 105:334–337.

76. Klepstad P, Rakvåg TT, Kaasa S, et al. The 118 A >G polymorphism in the human micro-opioid receptor gene may increase morphine requirements in patients with pain caused by malignant disease. Acta Anaesthesiol Scand 2004; 48:1232–1239.

77. Lötsch J, Skarke C, Wieting J, et al. Modulation of the central nervous effects of levomethadone by genetic polymorphisms potentially affecting its metabolism, distribution, and drug action. Clin Pharmacol Ther 2006; 79:72–89.

78. Ross JR, Rutter D, Welsh K, et al. Clinical response to morphine in cancer patients and genetic variation in candidate genes. Pharmacogenomics 2005; 5:324–336.

79. Zubieta JK, Heitzeg MM, Smith YR, et al. COMT val158met genotype affects mu-opioid neurotransmitter responses in pain stressor. Science 2003; 299:1240–1243.

80. Diatchenko L, Slade GD, Nackley AG, et al. Genetic basis for individual variations in pain perception and the development of a chronic pain condition. Hum Mol Genet 2005; 14:135–143.

81. Rakvag TT, Klepstad P, Baar C, et al. The Val158Met polymorphism of the human catechol-O-methyltransferase (COMT) gene mat influence morphine requirements in cancer pain patients. Pain 2005; 116:73–78.

82. Bernard S, Bruera E. Drug interactions in palliative care. J Clin Oncol 2000; 18: 1780–1799.

83. Crews JC, Sweeney NJ, Denson DD. Clinical efficacy of methadone in patients refractory to other mu-opioid receptor agonist analgesics for management of terminal cancer pain. Cancer 1993; 72:2266–2272.

84. Fallon M. Opioid rotation: does it have a role? Palliat Med 1997; 11:177–178.

85. Mercadante S, Casuccio A, Calderone L. Rapid switching from morphine to methadone in cancer patients with poor response to morphine. J Clin Oncol 1999; 17:3307–3312.

86. Abbadie C, Pasternak GW. Differential in vivo internalization of MOR-1 and MOR-1C by morphine. Neuroreport 2001; 12:3069–3072.

87. Pasternak DA, Pan L, Xu J, et al. Identification of three alternatively spliced variants of the rat mu opioid receptor gene: dissociation of affinity and efficacy. J Neurochem 2004; 91:881–890.

88. McMunnigall F, Welsh J. Opioid withdrawal syndrome on switching from hydro-morphone to alfentanil. Palliat Med 2008; 22(2):191–192.

89. Hanks GW, de Conno F, Cherny N, et al. Morphine and alternative opioids in cancer pain: the EAPC recommendations. Br J Cancer 2001; 84:1695–1700.

90. Kefalianakis F, Kugler M, van der Auwera R, et al. Die Opioid Rotation in der Schmerztherapie. Anaesthesist 2002; 51:28–32.

91. Indelicato RA, Portenoy RK. Opioid rotation in the management of refractory cancer pain. J Clin Oncol 2002; 20:348–352.

92. Anderson R, Saiers JH, Abram S, et al. Accuracy in equianalgesic dosing: conversion dilemmas. J Pain Symptom Manage 2001; 21(5):397–406.

93. Wedam EF, Bigelow GE, Johnson RE, et al. QT-interval effects of methadone, levomethadyl, and buprenorphine in a randomized trial. Arch Intern Med 2007; 167 (22):2469–2475.

94. Bruera E, Sweeney C. Methadone use in cancer patients with pain: a review. J Palliat Med 2002; 5:127–138.

95. Bruera E, Watanabe S, Fainsinger RL, et al. Custom-made capsules and suppositories of methadone for patients on high-dose opioids for cancer pain. Pain 1995; 62(2):141–146.

96. Lawlor PG, Turner KS, Hanson J, et al. Dose ratio between morphine and methadone in patients with cancer pain. Cancer 1998; 82(6):1167–1173.

97. Mercadante S, Bianchi M, Villari P, et al. Opioid plasma concentration during switching from morphine to methadone: preliminary data. Support Care Cancer 2003; 11(5):326–331.

98. Mercadante S, Casuccio A, Fulfaro F, et al. Switching from morphine to methadone to improve analgesia and tolerability in cancer patients: a prospective study. J Clin Oncol 2001; 19(11):2898–2904.

99. Morley JS, Watt JWG, Wells JC, et al. Methadone in pain uncontrolled by morphine. Lancet 1993; 342(81):1243.

100. Nauck F, Ostgathe C, Dickerson EDA. German model for methadone conversion. Am J Hosp Palliat Care 2001; 18(3):200–202.

101. Ripamonti C, De Conno F, Groff L, et al. Equianalgesic dose/ratio between methadone and other opioid agonists in cancer pain: comparison of two clinical experiences. Ann Oncol 1998; 9(1):79–83.

102. Ripamonti C, Groff L, Brunelli C, et al. Switching from morphine to oral methadone in treating cancer pain: what is the equianalgesic dose ratio? J Clin Oncol 1998; 16(10):3216–3221.

103. Scholes CF, Gonty N, Trotman IF. Methadone titration in opioid-resistant cancer pain. Eur J Cancer Care 1999; 8(1):26–29.

104. Weschules DJ, Bain KT. A systematic review of opioid conversion ratios used with methadone for the treatment of pain. Pain Med 2008; 9(5):595–612.

105. Wheeler W, Dickerson E. Clinical applications of methadone. Am J Hosp Palliat Care 2000; 17(3):196–203.

106. Davis M, Walsh D. Methadone for relief of cancer pain: a review of pharmacokinetics, pharmacodynamics, drug interactions and protocols of administration. Support Care Cancer 2001; 9(2):73–83.

107. Layson-Wolf C, Goode JV, Small RE. Clinical use of methadone. J Pain Palliat Care Pharmacother 2002; 16(1):29–59.

108. Fishman SM, Wilsey B, Mahajan G, et al. Methadone reincarnated: novel clinical applications with related concerns. Pain Med 2002; 3(4):339–348.
109. Manfredi PL, Houde RW. Prescribing methadone, a unique analgesic. J Support Oncol 2003; 1(3):216–220.
110. Soares L. Methadone for cancer pain: what have we learned from clinical studies? Am J Hosp Palliat Med 2005; 22(3):223–227.
111. Toombs JD, Kral LA. Methadone treatment for pain states. Am Fam Physician 2005; 71(7):1353–1358.
112. Manfredonia JF. Prescribing methadone for pain management in end-of-life care. J Am Osteopath Assoc 2005; 105(suppl 3):18S–21S.
113. Gordon DB, Stevenson KK, Grieffie J, et al. Opioid equianalgesic calculations. J Palliat Med 1999; 2(2):209–218.
114. Gammaitoni A, Fine P, Alvarez N, et al. Clinical application of opioid equianalgesic data. Clin J Pain 2003; 19(5):286–297.
115. Jacox A, Carr DB, Payne R, et al. Management of cancer pain. Clinical guideline number 9. Rockville, MD: Agency for Health Care Policy and Research, U.S. Department of Health and Human Services, Public Health Service; 1994. Report no.: AHCPR Publication No. 94–0592.
116. Rapp CJ, Gordon DB. Understanding equianalgesic dosing. Orthop Nurs 2000; 19 (3):65–70.
117. Brant JM. Opioid equianalgesic conversion: the right dose. Clin J Oncol Nurs 2001; 5(4):163–165.
118. FDA. Patient information: Duragesic® (fentanyl transdermal system). Manufactured by ALZA Corporation; Distributed by Janssen Pharmaceutica Products, L.P. 2003.
119. Levy M. Pharmacologic management of cancer pain. Semin Oncol 1994; 21(6): 718–739.
120. Donner B, Zenz M, Tryba M, Strumpf M. Direct conversion from oral morphine to transdermal fentanyl: a multicenter study in patients with cancer pain. Pain 1996; 64 (3):527–534.
121. Mercadante S, Ferrera P, Villar P, et al. Rapid switching between transdermal fentanyl and methadone in cancer patients. J Clin Oncol 2005; 23:5229–5234.
122. Hernansanz S, Gutiérrez C, Rubiales AS, et al.. Opioid rotation to methadone at home. J Pain Symptom Manage 2006; 31(1):2–4.
123. Bruera E, Pereira J, Watanabe S, et al. Opioid rotation in patients with cancer pain. A retrospective comparison of dose ratios between methadone, hydromorphone, and morphine. Cancer 1996; 78:852–857.
124. Morley JS, Makin MK. The use of methadone in cancer pain poorly responsive to other opioids. Pain Rev 1998; 5:51–58.
125. Morita T, Takigawa C, Onishi H, et al. Opioid rotation from morphine to fentanyl in delirious cancer patients: an open-label trial. J Pain Symptom Manage 2005; 30: 96–103.
126. Staats PS, Markowita J, Schein J. Incidence of constipation associated with long-acting opioid therapy: a comparative study. South Med J 2004; 97:129–134.
127. van Seventer R, Smit JM, Schipper RM, et al. Comparison of TTS-fentanyl with sustained-release oral morphine in the treatment of patients not using opioids for mild-to-moderate pain. Curr Med Res Opin 2003; 19:457–468.

128. Allan L, Richarz U, Simpson K, et al. Transdermal fentanyl sustained release oral morphine in strong-opioid naïve patients with chronic back pain. Spine 2005; 30:2484–2490.

129. Tarcatu D, Tamasdan C, Moryl N, et al. Are we still scratching the surface? A case of intractable pruritus following systemic opioid analgesia. J Opioid Mang 2007; 3(3):167–170.

130. Mercadante S, Willari P, Ferra P, et al. Opioid plasma concentrations during a switch from transdermal fentanyl to methadone. J Palliat Med 2007; 10(2):338–344.

131. Wirz S, Wartenberg HC, Elsen C, et al. Managing cancer pain and symptoms of outpatients by rotation to sustained-release hydromorphone: a prospective clinical trial. Clin J Pain 2006; 22(9):770–775.

132. Akiyama Y, Iseki M, Izawa R, et al. Usefulness of fentanyl patch (Durotep) in cancer patients when rotated from morphine preparations. Masui 2007; 56(3):317–323.

133. Narabayashi M, Saijo Y, Takenoshita S, et al. Opioid rotation from oral morphine to oral oxycodone in cancer patients with intolerable adverse effects: an open-label trial. Jpn J Clin Oncol 2008; 38(4):296–304.

134. McQuay H. Opioids in pain management. Lancet 1999; 353:2229–2232.

135. Kalso E, Heiskanen T, Rantio M, et al. Epidural and subcutaneous morphine in the management of cancer pain: a double-blind cross-over study. Pain 1996; 67:443–449.

136. Enting R, Oldenmenger W, van der Rijt C, et al. A prospective study evaluating the response of patients with unrelieved cancer pain to parenteral opioids. Cancer 2002; 94:3049–3056.

137. McCaffery M., Beebe A. Pain: Clinical Manual for Nursing Practice. St. Louis, MO: Mosby, 1989.

138. Anand KJS, Arnold JH. Opioid tolerance and dependence in infants and children. Pediatric Critical Care 1994; 22:334–342.

139. Foley KM, Inturrisi CE. Analgesic drug therapy in cancer pain: principles and practice. Med Clin North Am 1987; 71:207–232.

140. Parran L, Pederson C. Effects of an opioid taper algorithm in hematopoietic progenitor cell transplant recipients. Oncol Nurs Forum 2002; 29(1):41–50.

141. Berde C, Ablin A, Glazer J, et al. Report on the sub-committee on disease-related pain in childhood cancer. Pediatrics 1990; 86:818–825.

142. Anand KJS, Ingraham J. Tolerance, dependence, and strategies for compassionate withdrawal of analgesics and anxiolytics in the pediatric ICU. Critical Care Nurse 1996; 16(6):87–93.

143. Tzabazis AZ, Koppert W. Opioid-induced hyperalgesia or opioid-withdrawal hyperalgesia? Eur J Anesthesiol 2007; 24(9):811–820.

144. Wesson DR, Ling W. The clinical opiate withdrawal scales (COWS). J Psychoactive Drugs 2003; 35(2):253–259.

145. Amass L, Kamien JB, Mikulich SK. Efficacy of daily and alternate-day dosing regimens with the combinatïon buprenorphine–naloxone tablet. Drug Alcohol Depend 2000; 58:143–152.

146. Handelsman L, Cochrane KJ, Aronson MJ, et al. Two new rating scales for opioid withdrawal. Am J Drug Alcohol Abuse 1987; 13:293–308.

147. Gossop M. The development of a short opiate withdrawal scale (SOWS). Addict Behav 1990; 15(5):487–490.

148. Lawrinson P, Ali R, Buavirat A, et al. Key findings from the WHO collaborative study on subsitution therapy for opioid dependence and HIV/AIDS. Addiction 2008; 103(9):1484–1492.

149. Jang S, Kim H, Kim D, et al. Attenuation of morphine tolerance and withdrawal syndrome by coadministration of nalbuphine. Arch Pharm Res 2006; 29(8):677–684.

150. Lofwall MR, Walsh SL, Bigelow GE, et al. Modest opioid withdrawal suppression efficacy of oral tramadol in humans. Psychopharmacology (Berlin) 2007; 194(3): 381–393.

151. Gowing L, Farrell M, Ali R, et al. Alpha2 adrenergic agonists for the management of opioid withdrawal. Cochrane Database Syst Rev 2004; (4):CD002024.

152. McCambridge J, Gosspo M, Beswick T, et al. In-patient detoxification procedures, treatment retention, and post-treatment opiate use: comparison of lofexidine + naloxone, lofexidine + placebo, and methadone. Drug Alcohol Depend 2007; 88 (1):91–95.

153. Lin SK, Chen CH, Pan CH. Venlafxine for acute heroin detoxification: a double-blind, randomized, control trial. J Clin Psychopharmacol 2008; 28(2):189–194.

154. Freye E, Levy JV, Partecke L. Use of gabapentin for attenuation of symptoms following rapid opiate detoxification (ROD)-correlation with neurophysiological parameters. Neurophysiol Clin 2004; 34(2):81–90.

155. Zullino DF, Krenz S, Zimmerman G, et al. Topiramate in opiate withdrawal-comparison with clonidine and with carbamzepine/mianserin. Subst Abus 2004; 25(4):27–33.

156. Zullino DF, Krenz S, Favrat B, et al. The efficiency of a carbamazepine-mianserin combination scheme in opiate detoxification. Hum Psychopharmacol 2004; 19(6): 425–430.

157. Bexis S, Ong J, White J. Attenuation of morphine withdrawal signs by the GABA (B) receptor agonist baclofen. Life Sci 2001; 70(4):395–401.

158. Liu TT, Shi J, Epstein DH, et al. A meta-analysis of Chinese herbal medicine in treatment of managed withdrawal from heroin. Cell Mol Neurobiol 2009; 29(1):17–25.

159. Skelton KH, Oren D, Gutman DA, et al. The CRF1 receptor antagonist, R121919, attenuates the severity of precipitated morphine withdrawal. Eur J Pharmacol 2007; 571(1):17–24.

160. Kalange AS, Kokare DM, Singru PS, et al. Central administration of selective melanocotin 4 receptor antagonist HS014 prevents morphine tolerance and withdrawal hyperalgesia. Brain Res 2007; 1181:10–20.

161. Rehni AK, Bhateja P, Singh TG, et al. Nuclear factor-kappa-B inhibitor modulates the development of opioid dependence in a mouse model of naloxone-induced opioid withdrawal syndrome. Behav Pharmacol 2008; 19(3):265–269.

# 11

# Role of Adjuvant Medications in Managing Opioid-Induced Hyperalgesia

**David Giampetro and Yakov Vorobeychik**

*Department of Anesthesiology, Penn State Milton S. Hershey Medical Center, Penn State College of Medicine, Hershey, Pennsylvania, U.S.A.*

## INTRODUCTION

As a clinical entity, opioid-induced hyperalgesia (OIH) presents as pain not responding to, or worsening with, increasing doses of opioids. Hyperalgesia, allodynia, and the development of new areas of pain further suggest this disorder. The differential diagnosis and evaluation for this scenario have been discussed previously. Once it seems likely that OIH is present, treatment is centered on carefully decreasing the opioid dosing, also described previously. Other treatment options include the utilization of adjuvant medications and opioid rotation, which can be used preemptively or therapeutically (1,2).

## RATIONALE

As part of the strategy that utilizes more than one pain medication in a clinical regimen, opioid rotation and adjuvant medications are typically indicated in patients who are no longer responding to their opioid regimen or who develop intolerable side effects to their medications (3). The approach to switching from one opioid to another has been described in various reports and these serve as a guideline to accomplishing a switch. In cases of OIH, opioid rotation can be attempted as well and success with this approach has been described in the literature (4–7). The readers can find a detailed discussion on the issue of opioid rotation in a separate chapter by Dr Smith.

Rotation to different opioids provides an opportunity to decrease the opioid load due to decreased tolerance or OIH, especially when converting across different chemical categories such as from a phenanthrene (morphine) to a diphenylhaptane (methadone). It also provides opportunity to convert away from opioids like fentanyl and morphine that might be more likely to lead to OIH (8). Finally, rotating to methadone is an attractive option given that this chemical's D-isomer has *N*-methyl-D-aspartic acid (NMDA) receptor antagonistic properties. In fact, the majority of cases where opioid switching has worked have been with methadone.

Converting between opioids can be a challenge and physicians are often uncertain about this undertaking, especially when dealing with high doses of narcotic analgesics. The potency of a particular opioid on an individual is variable due to various biologic factors (9). Thus, the final dose of the target opioid is not absolutely predictable. It may be necessary to perform a rotation in a monitored setting if higher doses are involved and a rapid switch is desired, as may be the case in OIH where the pain is likely significant. Conversion tables can be used as an approximate guide only in performing an opioid rotation (Table 1). In cases of OIH it is possible to decrease the dose further than the conversion table suggests, i.e., under-dosing of the target opioid, as opposed to conventional opioid switching which is most commonly done for intolerable side effects of a particular opioid.

Ratios for switching between opioids have been investigated (3). Most reports are with respect to the conversion between morphine and another opioid. Thus, when converting between two opioids, neither of which is morphine, the conversion is based on their observed ratio with morphine in most cases. Guidelines from these reports are available and are reflected in the table. They are not absolute and variability is likely. The ratios also may not be the same in both directions. Switching from morphine to hydromorphone seems to be predictable at a ratio of 5:1 (morphine:hydromorphone) (10). Going from hydromorphone to morphine, interestingly, is slightly different, with a ratio closer to 1:4 (hydromorphone:morphine) (11). Since hydromorphone has a 3-glucuronide metabolite like morphine, it has potential neurotoxic effects. Oxycodone, on the other hand, does not possess such metabolites and may be more attractive if one is concerned about OIH. In such cases, conversion ratios may be approximately 1.4:1 (morphine:oxycodone) (12,13). This ratio applies to either direction of rotation.

Please note that approximately 10% of patients are poor metabolizers of oxycodone to its active metabolite, oxymorphone, and will require higher doses for conversion. Switching from morphine to transdermal fentanyl can be accomplished using a ratio of 100:1 (morphine:fentanyl) as a starting point, though a final ratio of 70–90:1 has been commonly observed (14–17). Of potential significance, one should note that the manufacturer's recommendation

**Table 1**  Opioid Conversion Guide

| Opioid | PO | IV | Sublingual | Transdermal | Comments |
|---|---|---|---|---|---|
| Morphine | 30 mg | 10 mg | – | – | – |
| Hydromorphone | 7.5 mg | 1.5 mg | – | – | – |
| Oxycodone | 20 mg | – | – | – | Variable reports, some use 1:1 conversion |
| Fentanyl | – | 0.1 mg | 0.1 mg | 12 µg/hr | |
| Methadone | Variable | – | – | – | See text |
| Oxymorphone | 10 mg | 1 mg | – | – | – |
| Hydrocodone | 20–60 mg | – | – | – | No accepted conversion |
| Propoxyphene | 130–200 mg | – | – | – | – |
| Codeine | 200 mg | – | – | – | – |
| Tramadol | 120 mg | – | – | – | – |
| Meperidine | 300 mg | 75 mg | – | – | Not recommended in chronic use |

This table is to be used as a guideline only. Final conversion ratios should be determined on a case-by-case basis. Variable patient responses are likely. Closely monitor patients during all conversions.

is 150:1, and that these ratios are for the total daily dose whereas the table describes conversion between total daily dose of morphine and µg/hr of fentanyl, as the patches are formulated and prescribed in this manner.

## Methadone

As suggested earlier, rotating to methadone is mechanistically appealing because the D-isomer of methadone is a weak NMDA-receptor antagonist, as well as a weak reuptake inhibitor of 5-hydroxytryptamine and norepinephrine. As detailed elsewhere in this book, the NMDA receptor plays a significant role in the development of OIH. Most of the reports in the literature detailing successful rotation of opioids in OIH use methadone as the target opioid (4–7). Not all conversions will result in success, but it is an endeavor worth trying if a patient is to remain on opioids. Switching to methadone has been the subject of many investigations and considerable concern due to the prolonged half-life of its metabolites and possibility for delayed toxicity.

Methadone undergoes biphasic elimination (18). The first phase is 8 to 12 hours and correlates with the analgesic effect. The second phase is 30 to 60 hours, and corresponds to the metabolites that limit withdrawal symptoms and can accumulate over time, leading to the delayed toxicity. Titration or conversion is thus advisable over a period of days to weeks. It is not advised to titrate methadone doses any more frequently than every fifth day in an outpatient setting, and these authors advise a protocol no sooner than every two weeks (18). With inpatients in a monitored setting, the conversion can be done more aggressively.

Needless to say, converting to methadone can be a difficult task. Switching to methadone from morphine is further complicated by a variable ratio depending on the starting dose of morphine. The ratio morphine:methadone has been observed to be anywhere between 3:1 and 20:1 (19–26). It seems that higher morphine doses require relatively less methadone. This certainly is in keeping with our current understanding of OIH, morphine toxicity, and methadone's opiate sparing effects. The median ratio observed is typically between 7:1 and 12:1. Given this variability, and the goal of a relative dose reduction in the case of OIH, the authors convert morphine to methadone at an initial ratio of 10:1 for up to 100 mg/day of morphine, 20:1 for doses above 300 mg/day, and about a 15:1 ratio between 100 and 300 mg/day of morphine. Conversion from hydromorphone is not well described. A conversion ratio for subcutaneous hydromorphone to oral methadone has been reported as 0.95:1 and 1.6:1 (subcutaneous hydromorphone:methadone) for patients receiving less than 330 mg hydromorphone per day and more than 330 mg/day, respectively (10). Given a 5:1 oral to parenteral equianalgesic ratio for hydromorphone, this would convert to an oral hydromorphone to oral methadone ratio of about 5:1 for typical doses of oral hydromorphone (27). A transdermal fentanyl to methadone ratio has been reported at 1:17 (28). This appears to be linear in relation to the fentanyl dose.

## BUPRENORPHINE AND OPIOID ANTAGONISTS

Though not advisable to employ in a conventional opioid rotation, partial opioid agonists like buprenorphine might be potentially effective in cases of OIH. Buprenorphine is a partial μ-opioid receptor agonist that, unlike pure μ-agonists, exerted a lasting inhibitory effect on secondary mechanical hyperalgesia in human volunteers with an intradermal electrical stimulation pain model (29). Partial agonists can induce withdrawal if given concomitantly with high doses of agonists, so that stronger opioids must be weaned to low doses before attempting to administer this type of medication. Likewise, ultra low doses of opioid receptor antagonists may be useful in OIH. They have been shown to potentiate the analgesic effect of conventional opioids, inhibit or reverse tolerance, and lessen side effects when used in combination with typical opioids (30). In the case of OIH, they may be useful in combinations or even as isolated agents. Naloxone is not a practical option because of its limited oral bioavailability. Naltrexone would be the best medication for outpatient use, but it is not available in ultra low-dose formulations. It has been reported that dissolution of the tablet in water has allowed administration of 1 to 5 μg/day (31). A combination of oxycodone and ultra low-dose naltrexone has been developed and may be useful in OIH. It has been shown to prolong analgesia and diminish dependence and tolerance, putatively via prevention of G-protein alterations involved in the development of tolerance and hyperalgesia (32,33).

## OTHER ADJUVANT MEDICATIONS

Numerous adjuvant medications are available in the treatment of pain, especially neuropathic type pain. Based on the understanding of pathophysiology of OIH and some similarities between neuropathic pain models and OIH, it is believed that adjuvant medications could be useful in the management and possibly in the prevention of this condition. Literature regarding these agents is limited, and those having been studied specifically in relation to OIH or having mechanisms that should affect OIH based on our current understanding of its development will be discussed further.

### NMDA-Receptor Antagonists

Perhaps the best-studied mechanistic aspect of OIH is the role of the NMDA receptor. It is not a surprise, then, that NMDA-receptor antagonists (NMDARA) have garnered a lot of attention in the management of OIH. Ketamine is discussed elsewhere. Other NMDRA include methadone, discussed earlier, as well as dextromethorphan, amantadine, and memantine (1). Dextromethorphan is a noncompetitive NMDARA used most commonly as a cough suppressant. Literature is mixed as to the utility of this agent in treating OIH or limiting tolerance (34,35). It may be that very high doses of dextromethorphan are required to achieve clinically relevant NMDARA effect needed to achieve these ends.

Amantadine has been used predominantly for its antiviral and antiparkinsonian effects. It has various mechanisms of action, including a noncompetitive antagonism of the NMDA receptor. A recent report demonstrated a decrease in morphine consumption and a lower visual analogue scale (VAS) pain scores in patients undergoing radical prostatectomy who received oral amantadine before and after surgery when compared to those who did not (36). This would suggest a possible role in decreasing opioid tolerance and OIH. Memantine is a derivative of amantadine that has been used primarily in the treatment of Alzheimer's disease. It has been shown to reduce hyperalgesia in animal models (37–39). Clinical evidence is mixed. A recent case series report of six patients with upper extremity complex regional pain syndrome (CRPS) who took memantine for six months demonstrated improved pain among other markers of disease, including functional MRI changes (40). Other studies have failed to demonstrate any effect of memantine on pain severity in various neuropathic pain states (41–44).

Magnesium has been proven to exert a noncompetitive voltage-dependent block of the NMDA receptor-operated ion channel, preventing extracellular calcium from entering the cell. It has been shown to enhance opioid analgesic affect and its deficiency has been implicated in inducing hyperalgesia that was reversible by an NMDA antagonist. (45,46). The opioid-sparing effect of magnesium may be greater at higher pain intensities and with increased dosages (47). Other studies examining magnesium failed to demonstrate preventive analgesia (48).

## Ca$^{2+}$ Channel Blockers

Gabapentin and pregabalin have been useful in numerous neuropathic pain states and also as adjuncts in epilepsy. These agents bind the $\alpha$-2 $\delta$-1 subunit of spinal voltage-gated calcium channels, possibly modulating the release of neurotransmitters involved on pain transmission and epileptogenesis. A recent animal study demonstrated that gabapentin, administered intrathecally may be effective in preventing OIH (49). In the study, rats were made hyperalgesic by subcutaneous injection of fentanyl. Following a brief increase in threshold to paw-pressure testing, the rats developed a delayed decrease in this nociceptive threshold, hence the development of hyperalgesia. Administration of gabapentin by either intrathecal or intraperitoneal route prevented this delayed hyperalgesic response in a dose-dependant fashion.

L-type calcium channel blockers such as nifedipine may play a role in treating of OIH as well. It has been shown that opioid receptors interact with L-type calcium channels and this interaction may allow for prolonged action potential duration due to increase in calcium channel currents (50). In a recent study, low-dose morphine was used to induce hyperalgesia in rats as assessed by a tail-flick latency test. Intrathecal administration of nifedipine completely blocked the hyperalgesic effect (50). The authors propose several possible mechanisms for this, including increased intracellular calcium, inhibition of morphine-induced cholecystokinin (CCK) release at the dorsal horn, and inhibition of NMDA-receptor function.

## Miscellaneous Adjuvant Medications

Prostaglandins have been implicated in pronociception and cyclooxygenase (COX) inhibitors demonstrated an ability to block hyperalgesia and reverse opioid tolerance in rats (1). Thus, it is likely that COX inhibitors will be of benefit in managing OIH. Little human data in cases of OIH has been known. Parecoxib, a COX-2 inhibitor, has been shown to decrease remifentanil-induced hyperalgesia in an intradermal electrical stimulation pain model if administered prior to opioid exposure (51). Similarly, $\alpha$-2 adrenergic agonists may be useful in OIH. It has been demonstrated that clonidine administration can lessen post opioid infusion anti-analgesia and secondary hyperalgesia (1).

Proglumide is a CCK antagonist originally employed in the treatment of peptic ulcers. It is not readily available because its role in ulcer treatment has become obsolete. It has been suggested that CCK is involved in the development of OIH and tolerance. The rostral ventromedial medulla (RVM) is the source of a descending pain facilitation pathway to the dorsal horn via the dorsolateral fasciculus (DLF). Lidocaine administration into the RVM or lesioning of the DLF has been shown to reverse OIH in animals (52). It is further demonstrated that CCK may be the chemical messenger in the RVM that drives this mechanism (52). Blockade of the CCK-2 receptors in the RVM of rats reversed morphine-induced hyperalgesia. Proglumide has been shown to enhance analgesic efficacy of morphine and dihydrocodeine (53,54). It has not been assessed in OIH to date.

Buspirone is a 5-hydroxytryptamine 1A (5HT$_{1A}$) receptor agonist used in the treatment of anxiety. No evidence has been put forth showing any utility in OIH or tolerance, but there is evidence that 5HT$_{1A}$ excitation causes hyperalgesia followed by analgesia, in a similar phenomenological mechanism to OIH but in the opposite direction (55). There have been no studies to date using the experimental 5HT$_{1A}$ agonists to reverse OIH in animals or humans, but it has been demonstrated that continued application of a 5HT$_{1A}$ agonist (F13640) for two weeks in a rat model of spinal cord injury led to significant analgesia (56).

## CONCLUSION

Numerous pathophysiological mechanisms have been implicated in OIH, and the attempts to treat this condition using a mechanistic approach have started just recently. Hopefully, continuous focus of future investigations on solving this problem will improve the quality of life of many patients with intractable opioid-resistant pain.

## REFERENCES

1. Chu LF, Angst MS, Clark D. Opioid induced hyperalgesia in humans: molecular mechanisms and clinical considerations. Clin J Pain 2008; 24(6):479–496.
2. Chang G, Chen L, Mao J. Opioid tolerance and hyperalgesia. Med Clin N Am 2007; 91:199–211.
3. Mecandante S, Bruera B. Opioid switching: a systematic and critical review. Cancer Treat Rev 2006; 32:304–315.
4. Vorobeychik Y, Chen L, Chasko Bush M, et al. Improved analgesic effect following opioid dose reduction. Pain Med 2008; 9(6):724–727.
5. Axelrod DJ, Reville B. Using methadone to treat opioid-induced hyperalgesia and refractory pain. J Opioid Manage 2007; 3(2):113–114.
6. Mercandate S, Arcuri E. Hyperalgeisa and opioid switching. Am J Hosp Palliat Care 2005; 22:291–294.
7. Chung KS, Carson S, Glassman D, et al. Successful treatment of hydromorphone induced neurotoxicity and hyperalgesia. Conn Med 2004; 68:547–549.
8. Zylicz Z, Twycross R. Opioid induced hyperalgesia may be more frequent than previously thought (correspondence). J Clin Oncol 2008; 26(9):1564.
9. Mercandate S. Opioid rotation for cancer pain. Rationale and clinical aspects. Cancer 1999; 86:1856–1866.
10. Bruera E, Pereira J, Watanabe S, et al. Opioid rotation in patients with cancer pain. A retrospective comparison of dose ratios between methadone, hydromorphone, and morphine. Cancer 1996; 78:852–857.
11. Lawlor P, Turner K, Hanson J, et al. Dose ratio between morphine and hydromorphone in patients with cancer pain: a retrospective study. Pain 1997; 72:79–85.

12. Maddocks I, Somogyi A, Abbott F, et al. Attenuation of morphine-induced delirium in palliative care by substitution with infusion of oxycodone. J Pain Symptom Manage 1996; 12:182–189.

13. Gagnon B, Bielech M, Watanabe S, et al. The use of intermittent subcutaneous injections of oxycodone for opioid rotation in patients with cancer pain. Support Care Cancer 1999; 7:265–270.

14. Donner B, Zenz M, Tryba M, et al. Direct conversion from oral morphine to transdermal fentanyl: a multicenter study in patients with cancer pain. Pain 1996; 64:527–534.

15. Morita T, Takigawa C, Onishi H, et al. Opioid rotation from morphine to fentanyl in delirious cancer patients: an open-label trial. J Pain Symptom Manage 2005; 30:96–103.

16. Watanabe S, Pereira J, Hanson J, et al. Fentanyl by continuous subcutaneous infusion for the management of cancer pain: a retrospective study. J Pain Symptom Manage 1998; 16:323–326.

17. Paix A, Coleman K, Less, J, et al. Subcutaneous fentanyl and sufentanil infusion substitution for morphine intolerance in cancer pain management. Pain 1995; 63: 263–269.

18. Mahajan G, Fishman S. Major opioids in pain management. In: Benzon H, Raja S, Molloy R, et al., eds. Essentials of Pain Medicine and Regional Anesthesia. Philadelphia, PA: Elsevier, 2005:94–105.

19. Lawlor P, Turner K, Hanson J, et al. Dose ratio between morphine and methadone in patients with cancer pain. A retrospective study. Cancer 1998; 82:1167–1173.

20. Ripamonti C, Groff L, Brunelli C, et al. Switching from morphine to oral methadone in treating cancer pain: what is the equianalgesic ratio? J Clin Oncol 1998; 16:3216–3221.

21. Scholes C, Gonty N, Trotman L. Methadone titration in opioid-resistant cancer pain. Eur J Cancer Care 1999; 8:26–29.

22. Morlet JS, Wells JC, Miles JB. Methadone in pain uncontrolled by morphine. Lancet 1993; 342:1243.

23. Blackburn D, Somerville E, Squire J. Methadone: an alternative conversion regime. Eur J Palliat Care 2002; 9:92–96.

24. Mercandate S, Casussio A, Calderone L. Rapid switching from morphine to methadone in cancer patients with poor response to morphine. J Clin Oncol 1999; 17:3301–3312.

25. Mercandate S, Bianchi M, Villari P, et al. Opioid plasma concentration during switching from morphine to methadone: preliminary data. Support Care Cancer 2003; 11:326–331.

26. Trescot A, Datta S, Lee M, et al. Opioid pharmacology. Pain Physician 2008; 11(3): S133–S153.

27. Murray A, Hagen NA. Hydromorphone. J Pain Symptom Manage 2005; 29(5S):S57–S66.

28. Benitez-Rosario MA, Ferla M, Salinas-Martin A, et al. Opioid switching from transdermal fentanyl to oral methadone in patients with cancer pain. Cancer 2004; 101:2866–2873.

29. Koppert W, Ihmsen H, Korber N, et al. Different profiles of buprenorphine-induced analgesia and antihyperalgesia in a human pain model. Pain 2005; 118:15–22.

30. Holtsman M, Fishman S. Opioid receptors. In: Benzon H, Raja S, Molloy R, et al., eds. Essentials of Pain Medicine and Regional Anesthesia. Philadelphia, PA: Elsevier, 2005:94–105.

31. Zylicz Z, Krajnik M. Opioid-induced hyperalgesia as a problem in pain management. Mechanisms of onset, diagnosis, and treatment. Adv Palliat Med 2007; 6(1):37–44.

32. Chindalore VL, Craven RA, Yu KP, et al. Adding ultralow-dose naltrexone to oxycodone enhances and prolongs analgesia: a randomized, controlled trial of oxytrex. J Pain 2005; 6(6):392–399.
33. Webster LR, Butera PG, Moran LV, et al. Oxytrex minimizes physical dependence while providing effective analgesia: a randomized controlled trial in low back pain. J Pain 2006; 7(12):937–946.
34. Galer BS, Lee D, Ma T, et al. Morphidex (morphine sulfate/dextromethorphan hydrobromide combination) in the treatment of chronic pain: three multicenter, randomized, double-blind, controlled clinical trials fail to demonstrate enhanced opioid analgesia or reduction in tolerance. Pain 2005; 115:284–295.
35. Katz NP. Morphidex (MS:DM) double-blind, multiple-dose studies in chronic pain patients. J Pain Symptom Manage 2000; 19:S42–S49.
36. Snijdelaar DG, Koren G, Katz J. Effects of perioperative amantadine on postoperative pain and morphine consumption in patients after radical prostatectomy. Anesthesiology 2004; 100:134–141.
37. Eisenberg E, LaCross S, Strassman AM. The clinically tested $N$-methyl-D-aspartate receptor antagonist memantine blocks and reverses thermal hyperalgesia in a rat model of painful mononeuropathy. Neurosci Lett 1995; 187:17–20.
38. Carlton SM, Hargett GL. Treatment with the NMDA antagonist memantine attenuates nociceptive responses to mechanical stimulation in neuropathic rats. Neurosci Lett 1995; 198:115–118.
39. Chaplan SR, Malmberg AB, Yaksh TL. Efficacy of spinal NMDA receptor antagonism in formalin hyperalgesia and nerve injury evoked allodynia in the rat. J Pharmacol Exp Ther 1997; 280:829–838.
40. Sinis N, Birbaumer N, Gustin S, et al. Memantine treatment of complex regional pain syndrome: a preliminary report of six cases. Clin J Pain 2007; 23:237–243.
41. Schifitto G, Yiannoutsos CT, Simpson DM, et al. A placebo-controlled study of memantine for the treatment of human immunodeficiency virus-associated sensory neuropathy. J Neurovirol 2006; 12:328–331.
42. Sang CN, Booher S, Gilron I, et al. Dextromethorphan and memantine in painful diabetic neuropathy and postherpetic neuralgia: efficacy and dose-response trials. Anesthesiology 2002; 96:1053–1061.
43. Eisenberg E, Kleiser A, Dortort A, et al. The NMDA ($N$-methyl-D-aspartate) receptor antagonist memantine in the treatment of postherpetic neuralgia: a double-blind, placebo-controlled study. Eur J Pain 1998; 2:321–327.
44. Nikolajsen L, Gottrup H, Kristensen AG, et al. Memantine (a $N$-methyl-D-aspartate receptor antagonist) in the treatment of neuropathic pain after amputation or surgery: a randomized, double-blinded, cross-over study. Anesth Analg 2000; 91:960–966.
45. Begon S, Pickering G, Eschalier A, et al. Magnesium increases morphine analgesic effect in different experimental models of pain. Anesthesiology 2002; 96:627–632.
46. Dubray C, Alloui A, Bardin L, et al. Magnesium deficiency induces a hyperalgesia reversed by the NMDA receptor antagonist MK801. Neuroreport 1997; 8: 1383–1386.
47. Steinlechner B, Dworschak M, Birkenberg B, et al. Magnesium moderately decreases remifentanil dosage required for pain management after cardiac surgery. Br J Anaesth 2006; 96(4):444–449.

48. McCartney C, Sinha A, Katz, J. A qualitative systematic review of the role of *N*-methyl-D-aspartate antagonists in preventive analgesia. Anesth Analg 2004; 98(5): 1385–1400.

49. Van Elstraete AC, Sitbon P, Mazoit JP, et al. Gabapentin prevents delayed and long-lasting hyperalgesia induced by fentanyl in rats. Anesthesiology 2008; 108:484–494.

50. Esmaeili-Mahani S, Shimokawa N, Javan M, et al. Low-dose morphine induces hyperalgesia through activiation of $G_{\alpha s}$, protein kinase C, and L-type $Ca^{2+}$ channels in rats. J Neurosci Res 2008; 86:471–479.

51. Troster A, Sittl R, Singler B, et al. Modulation of remifentanil induced analgesia and postinfusion hyperalgesia by parecoxib in humans. Anesthesiology 2006; 105:1016–1023.

52. Xie JY, Herman DS, Stiller CO, et al. Cholecystokinin in the rostral ventromedial medulla mediates opioid-induced hyperalgesia and antinociceptive tolerance. J Neurosci 2005; 25(2):409–416.

53. McCleane GJ. The cholecystokinin antagonist proglumide enhances the analgesic efficacy of morphine in humans with chronic benign pain. Anesth Analg 1998; 87:1117–1120.

54. McCleane GJ. The cholecystokinin antagonist proglumide enhances the analgesic effect of dihydrocodeine. Clin J Pain 2003; 19:200–201.

55. Xu XJ, Colpaert F, Wiesenfeld-Hallin Z. Opioid hyperalgesia and tolerance versus 5-$HT_{1A}$ receptor-mediated inverse tolerance. Trends Pharmacol Sci 2003; 24(12): 634–639.

56. Deseure K. Continuous administration of the 5-$HT_{1A}$ agonist, F 13640, attenuates allodynia-like behavior in a rat model of trigeminal neuropathic pain. J Pharmacol Exp Ther 2003; 306:505–514.

# Clinical Implications of Opioid-Induced Hyperalgesia

Jianren Mao

*Department of Anesthesia, Critical Care, and Pain Medicine, Massachusetts General Hospital, Harvard Medical School, Boston, Massachusetts, U.S.A.*

## INTRODUCTION

Compelling evidence has accumulated over the past decade indicating that hyperalgesia may occur in the absence of an overt, precipitated withdrawal from opioid analgesics. This paradoxical opioid-induced hyperalgesia may be a contributing factor of apparent clinical opioid tolerance, referring to the need of dose escalation to maintain the opioid analgesic effect. Until recently, the diminished opioid analgesic effect during a course of opioid therapy is often attributed to the presence of pharmacological opioid tolerance (i.e., desensitization of the responsiveness of the opioid receptor and its cellular mechanism) and/or a worsening clinical pain condition. Accordingly, opioid dose escalation appears to be a logical approach to restoring the lost effectiveness of opioid analgesics. This practice should be reconsidered in light of information on opioid-induced hyperalgesia (1).

In the clinical setting, apparent opioid tolerance may result from pharmacological tolerance, worsening pain condition due to disease progression, and/or opioid-induced hyperalgesia (Fig. 1). Although the clinical presentation of apparent clinical opioid tolerance manifests as the diminished opioid analgesic effect, the approach to resolving this condition could be very different. For example, opioid dose escalation would be a logical clinical step to overcome

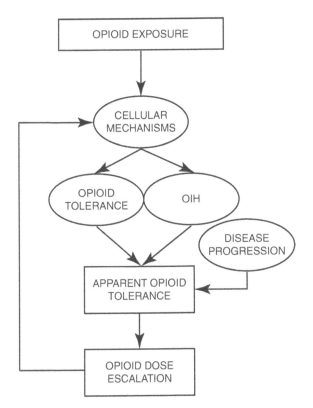

**Figure 1** Apparent clinical opioid tolerance may result from pharmacological tolerance, a worsening pain state due to disease progression, and/or opioid-induced hyperalgesia (OIH). Opioid dose escalation may overcome pharmacological tolerance and treat worsening pain conditions due to disease progression. However, opioid dose escalation may enhance the pronociceptive process and worsen apparent opioid tolerance and clinical pain due to the exacerbation of opioid-induced hyperalgesia. The clinical outcome depends on the balance between the opioid analgesic effect and opioid-induced hyperalgesic response.

pharmacological tolerance and worsening pain conditions due to disease progression, if there are no contraindications (e.g., the patient's tolerability to dose escalation). However, if opioid-induced hyperalgesia is the main cause of the lack of opioid analgesic effect because hyperalgesia counteracts this effect; opioid dose escalation could enhance the pronociceptive process, further worsening apparent opioid tolerance and clinical pain.

Therefore, a practical issue is how to distinguish opioid-induced hyperalgesia from a worsening pain state and opioid tolerance? In preceding chapters, details regarding the diagnosis of opioid-induced hyperalgesia and useful approaches to managing opioid-induced hyperalgesia have been discussed. In this final chapter, the clinical implications of opioid-induced hyperalgesia in opioid therapy will be summarized and future research directions will be discussed.

**Table 1** Differential Diagnosis of OIH

| Clinical factor | OIH | Opioid tolerance |
|---|---|---|
| Exacerbated temporal summation of second pain (QST) | Yes | No |
| Decreased pain threshold (QST) | Yes | No |
| Decreased pain tolerance (QST) | Yes | No |
| Relationship with opioid dose (the higher, the more likely to be present) | Yes | Yes |
| Relationship with duration of opioid treatment (the longer, the more likely to be present) | Yes | Yes |
| Opioid dose escalation | Limited improvement in clinical pain scale and QST responses | Improved pain relief |
| Opioid dose reduction | Improved opioid analgesia | Reduced opioid analgesia |
| Pain quality | Burning, diffuse pain, and spontaneous pain similar to those seen with neuropathic pain | No change |
| Pain location | At and/or beyond the dermatome distribution of a preexisting pain condition | No change |
| Pain intensity | Similar or greater than the preexisted pain condition | Similar to the preexisted pain condition |
| Influence by opioid type | Unclear | Unclear |
| Influence by gender | Unclear | Unclear |

*Abbreviations*: OIH, opioid-induced hyperalgesia; QST, quantitative sensory testing.

## DIFFERENTIAL DIAGNOSIS AND MANAGEMENT OF OPIOID-INDUCED HYPERALGESIA

Several categories of clinical factors could be considered in the differential diagnosis of opioid-induced hyperalgesia in a clinical setting (Table 1), which may include characteristic quantitative sensory testing (QST) responses, relevant clinical factors, changes in pain pattern and location, and other factors (e.g., gender, opioid type). Moreover, these clinical factors should be considered along with additional clinical information such as the use of adjunctive nonopioid pain medications and the presence of comorbidities.

1. Opioid-induced hyperalgesia would conceivably exacerbate a preexisted pain condition. For example, the overall pain intensity (e.g., on a visual analog scale) following opioid treatment would be increased above the level of preexisted pain in the absence of disease progression. Opioid dose

escalation only transiently and minimally reduces the pain intensity with a subsequent increase in the pain intensity.

2. The quality, location, and distribution pattern related to opioid-induced hyperalgesia would be different from preexisted pain condition. Because opioid analgesics are often administered systemically, such changes would be diffuse as compared to the preexisted pain condition. Since the mechanisms of opioid-induced hyperalgesia have many characteristics in common with the mechanisms of pathological pain such as neuropathic pain, changes in pain threshold, tolerability, and distribution patterns indicative of opioid-induced hyperalgesia would be similar to the features seen in neuropathic pain patients. Moreover, QST may be a useful tool to detect such changes (see the following section for more discussion).

3. When the differential diagnosis is uncertain, a trial of opioid dose escalation or decrease may be a helpful tool in the clinical setting. For example, the under-treated pain condition, a worsening pain condition due to disease progress, and/or pharmacological opioid tolerance may all be overcome by a trial of opioid dose escalation, whereas dose escalation may exacerbate opioid-induced hyperalgesia. In contrast, a supervised opioid tapering may reduce opioid-induced hyperalgesia and improve the clinical pain management. In this regard, if a patient is on a low opioid dose regimen and complains of unsatisfactory pain relief, a trial of opioid dose escalation may be appropriate. If a patient is already on very high doses of opioid analgesics, further dose escalation makes little sense and may just exacerbate opioid-induced hyperalgesia.

4. It is important to consider that the clinical outcome of an opioid therapy is a dynamic balance between the opioid analgesic effect and opioid hyperalgesic effect. Whenever there is an opioid dose escalation (enhancing the analgesic effect), it is always possible that the patient may transiently benefit from the dose escalation even if there exists opioid-induced hyperalgesia in the same patient. The issue is that the dose escalation would also exacerbate opioid-induced hyperalgesia, which may quickly overturn the transient increase in the opioid analgesic effect due to the dose escalation. In some cases, repeated opioid escalation becomes a futile process of transient pain relief followed by worsening pain. Therefore, clinical judgment is fundamentally important and, whenever a dose change (increase or decrease) is being contemplated, all clinical conditions related to opioid therapy need to be considered in the decision-making process.

## QST AS A DIAGNOSTIC TOOL FOR OPIOID-INDUCED HYPERALGESIA

As discussed in several chapters, QST is a useful tool to assess opioid-induced hyperalgesia. In a recent study (2), QST was used to compare pain threshold, pain tolerance, and the degree of temporal summation of the second pain in response to thermal stimulation among three groups of subjects: those with neither pain nor opioid therapy (group 1), those with chronic pain but without opioid therapy (group 2), and those with both chronic pain and opioid therapy (group 3). The possible correlation between QST responses to thermal stimulation and opioid dose, opioid treatment duration, opioid analgesic type, pain duration, or gender was also examined in group 3 subjects. As compared with both group 1 and group 2 subjects, group 3 subjects displayed a decreased heat pain threshold and exacerbated temporal summation of the second pain to thermal stimulation, and there were no differences in cold or warm sensation among all three groups.

Among clinical factors, daily opioid dose consistently correlated with the decreased heat-pain threshold and exacerbated temporal summation of the second pain in group 3 subjects. It is of interest to note that QST changes detected in chronic pain subjects with opioid therapy do not necessarily indicate that opioid-induced hyperalgesia has contributed to the clinical phenomenon of apparent opioid tolerance. What it does indicate is that these subjects have altered responses to a standard battery of noxious stimulation. These results indicate that decreased heat pain threshold and exacerbated temporal summation of the second pain may be characteristic QST changes in subjects with opioid therapy and suggest that QST may be a useful tool in the clinical assessment of opioid-induced hyperalgesia.

## INFLUENCE OF OPIOID REGIMEN ON OPIOID-INDUCED HYPERALGESIA

Opioid regimens may influence the development of opioid-induced hyperalgesia. For example, the development of opioid-induced hyperalgesia may differ based on the type and dose of opioid analgesics (e.g., morphine vs. methadone). Anecdotal clinical observations have indeed suggested that the degree of opioid-induced pain may vary according to opioid analgesics (3). While the exact temporal relationship between the dose regimen and the development of opioid-induced hyperalgesia remains to be determined, it is conceivable that opioid-induced pain would be more likely to develop in patients receiving high opioid doses with a prolonged treatment course, although opioid-induced hyperalgesia has been demonstrated in patients receiving a short course of highly potent opioid analgesics (4). Moreover, patients with a pathological pain condition (e.g., neuropathic pain) treated with opioid therapy may be more susceptible to developing opioid-induced hyperalgesia because both pathological pain and opioid-induced hyperalgesia may share a common cellular mechanism (5).

Is there cross pain sensitivity to different opioids? That is, if opioid-induced hyperalgesia develops following exposure to one opioid, can switching to a different opioid diminish opioid-induced hyperalgesia (6)? The lack of cross pain sensitivity between different opioids would be a beneficial factor in clinical opioid therapy. At least, incomplete tolerance to different opioids may be a good reason to switch between different opioids if there exists apparent clinical opioid tolerance, because an enhanced opioid analgesic effect through opioid rotation would counteract opioid-induced hyperalgesia regardless of whether the rotation itself reduces opioid-induced hyperalgesia.

## OPIOID-INDUCED HYPERALGESIA AND PREEMPTIVE ANALGESIA

Despite the ongoing debate on the clinical effectiveness of preemptive analgesia in pain management, the use of opioid analgesic as the sole agent for preemptive analgesia may not be desirable for several reasons. First, a large dose of intraoperative opioids could activate a pronociceptive mechanism leading to the development of postoperative opioid-induced hyperalgesia (7). This may confound the assessment of postoperative pain and counteract the opioid analgesic effect. Second, preemptive analgesia calls for preemptive inhibition of neural plastic changes mediated through multiple cellular mechanisms such as the central glutamatergic system. Paradoxically, opioid administration could activate the central glutamatergic system as discussed above (8,9). Third, neural mechanisms of opioid tolerance and opioid-induced hyperalgesia may interact with the mechanisms of pathological pain, whereas pathological pain could be exacerbated with opioid administration (8,9). Nonetheless, this issue needs to be investigated in future studies.

## UNRESOLVED ISSUES

Several issues may be considered in the direction of future research on opioid-induced hyperalgesia. For example, most clinical studies have used QST as a tool to assess opioid-induced hyperalgesia in human subjects. Despite the unique features of QST, it is sometimes difficult to compare pain intensity between groups (e.g., subjects with or without opioids) by using QST alone. Most preclinical studies of opioid-induced hyperalgesia were conducted in animals without a pathological pain condition, whereas in the clinical setting opioid analgesics are used for the pain management. Similarly, many human studies of opioid-induced hyperalgesia were conducted in subjects without clinical pain. This mismatch between preclinical and clinical conditions makes it difficult to fully assess the clinical impact of opioid-induced hyperalgesia in chronic opioid therapy. Furthermore, opioid analgesics have the addiction potential despite the legitimate medical use. Addiction to opioid analgesics in the setting of pain management raises another important scientific and clinical question, that is, would the addictive property of opioid analgesics interact with pain and alter clinical features of opioid-induced hyperalgesia?

## SUMMARY

Opioid-induced hyperalgesia should be considered when the adjustment of opioid dose is contemplated if (*i*) prior opioid dose escalation failed to provide the expected analgesic effect and (*ii*) there is unexplainable pain exacerbation following an initial period of effective opioid analgesia. Although in some cases increasing opioid dose leads to the improved pain management, in other cases less opioid may lead to more effective pain reduction. This goal may be accomplished by using opioid rotation, adding adjunctive medications, combining opioid with clinically available $N$-methyl-D-aspartate receptor antagonist, and/or initiating a trial of opioid tapering (1,5,8–12).

## REFERENCES

1. Mao J. Opioid-induced abnormal pain sensitivity—implications in clinical opioid therapy. Pain 2002; 100:213–217.
2. Chen L, Malarick C, Seefeld L, et al. Altered quantitative sensory testing outcome in subjects with opioid therapy. Pain 2009; 143:65–70.
3. Compton P, Charuvastra VC, Ling W. Pain intolerance in opioid-maintained former opiate addicts: effect of long-acting maintenance agent. Drug Alcohol Depend 2001; 63:139–146.
4. Vinik HR, Kissin I. Rapid development of tolerance to analgesia during remifentanil infusion in humans. Anesth Analg 1998; 86:1307–1311.
5. Mao J, Price DD, Mayer DJ. Mechanisms of hyperalgesia and opioid tolerance: a current view of their possible interactions. Pain 1995; 62:259–274.
6. Sjogren P, Jensen NH, Jensen TS. Disappearance of morphine-induced hyperalgesia after discontinuing or substituting morphine with opioid agonists. Pain 1994; 59:313–316.
7. Guignard B, Bossard AE, Coste C, et al. Acute opioid tolerance: intraoperative remifentanil increases postoperative pain and morphine requirement. Anesthesiology 2000; 93:409–417.
8. Angst MS, Clark JD. Opioid-induced hyperalgesia: a qualitative systematic review. Anesthesiology 2006; 104:570–587.
9. Baron MJ, McDonald PW. Significant pain reduction in chronic pain patients after detoxification from high-dose opioids. J Opioid Manage 2006; 2:277–282.
10. Visser E, Schug SA. The role of ketamine in pain management. Biomed Pharmacother 2006; 60:341–348.
11. Van Elstraete AC, Sitbon P, Trabold F, et al. A single dose of intrathecal morphine in rats induces long-lasting hyperalgesia: the protective effect of prior administration of ketamine. Anesth Analg 2005; 101:1750–1756.
12. Ballantyne J, Mao J. Opioid therapy for chronic pain. New Engl J Med 2003; 349: 1943–1953.

# Index

Milton Keynes UK
Ingram Content Group UK Ltd.
UKHW022107141024
449569UK00031B/1817